WALKER'S EXERCISES FOR LA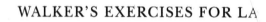

WALKER'S EXERCISES FOR LADIES

CALCULATED TO

PRESERVE AND IMPROVE BEAUTY

AND

TO PREVENT AND CORRECT PERSONAL DEFECTS

inseparable from constrained or careless habits

FOUNDED ON

Physiological Principles

BY DONALD WALKER

MICHAEL JOSEPH

AN IMPRINT OF
PENGUIN BOOKS

MICHAEL JOSEPH

UK | USA | Canada | Ireland | Australia
India | New Zealand | South Africa

Michael Joseph is part of the Penguin Random House group of companies
whose addresses can be found at global.penguinrandomhouse.com

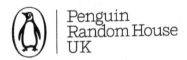

First published by Thomas Hurst 1834
This edition published by Michael Joseph 2018

001

Set in New Baskerville ITC Pro and Bulmer MT Pro
Typeset by Jouve (UK), Milton Keynes
Printed in Great Britain by Clays Ltd, St Ives plc

A CIP catalogue record for this book is available from the British Library

HARDBACK ISBN: 978–0–241–34916–8

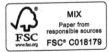

DEDICATION

CONTENTS

PECULIARITIES OF THE PRESENT SYSTEM · · · 1

PART I

REASONINGS ON WHICH ARE FOUNDED THE EXERCISES HERE EMPLOYED

OF THE STRUCTURE OF THE BODY AS CONNECTED
WITH EXERCISE 5
  Of the Body Generally 5
  Of the Vertebral Column in Particular . . . 6
  Important Circumstances to be Noted . . . 8

OF THE FUNCTIONS OF THE BODY AS AFFECTED
BY EXERCISE 10

OF THE CONSTRAINT TO WHICH THE BODY IS
WRONGLY SUBJECTED 15

OF THE DEBILITY WHICH IS CAUSED BY
CONSTRAINT 17

OF THE WRONG POSITIONS WHICH RESULT FROM
DEBILITY, AND FROM THE EMPLOYMENT, IN THE
PARTICULAR PURSUITS OF EDUCATION, OR THE
COMMON ACTS OF LIFE, OF MUSCLES
UNFAVOURABLY SITUATED   ·   ·   ·   ·   ·   ·   18

   In Standing   ·   ·   ·   ·   ·   ·   ·   ·   ·   19
   In Sitting ·   ·   ·   ·   ·   ·   ·   ·   ·   ·   19
   In Writing ·   ·   ·   ·   ·   ·   ·   ·   ·   22
   In Drawing   ·   ·   ·   ·   ·   ·   ·   ·   ·   22
   In Guitar-Playing   ·   ·   ·   ·   ·   ·   ·   25
   In Harp-Playing   ·   ·   ·   ·   ·   ·   ·   28
   In Riding   ·   ·   ·   ·   ·   ·   ·   ·   28
   In Lying in Bed ·   ·   ·   ·   ·   ·   ·   ·   31

OF THE DEFORMITY IN WHICH WRONG POSITIONS
TERMINATE   ·   ·   ·   ·   ·   ·   ·   ·   ·   ·   32

   The Injury thus Done to the Locomotive Organs
     and Functions, or those on which General Motion
     Depends·   ·   ·   ·   ·   ·   ·   ·   ·   ·   32
   The Injury thus Done to the Vital Organs and
     Functions, or those on which Life Depends   ·   ·   39
   The Injury thus Done to the Mental Organs and
     Functions, or those on which Thought Depends   ·   41

OF THE PARTICULAR AND SPECIAL UTILITY OF
EXERCISES   ·   ·   ·   ·   ·   ·   ·   ·   ·   ·   44

PART II

PARTICULAR EXERCISES

OF THE KINDS OF EXERCISE   ·   ·   ·   ·   ·   ·   51
PASSIVE EXERCISES ·   ·   ·   ·   ·   ·   ·   ·   52

MIXED EXERCISES · · · · · · · · · · 55
ACTIVE EXERCISES – OF POSITION · · · · 56
   Of Standing Generally · · · · · · · 56
   Fundamental Position · · · · · · · · 58
   Positions in Dancing · · · · · · · · 61
EXTENSION MOTIONS · · · · · · · · 64
THE EXERCISE WITH THE ROD · · · · · · 69
   First Exercise · · · · · · · · · · 69
   Second Exercise · · · · · · · · · 69
   Third Exercise · · · · · · · · · · 71
   Fourth Exercise · · · · · · · · · 71
THE DUMB-BELLS · · · · · · · · · 72
   First Exercise · · · · · · · · · · 72
   Second Exercise · · · · · · · · · 75
   Third Exercise · · · · · · · · · · 75
   Fourth Exercise · · · · · · · · · 75
THE INDIAN SCEPTRE EXERCISE · · · · · 76
   The Portion Practised with Clubs in the Army · · 76
   The New and More Beautiful Portion Now Added
     from the Indian Practice · · · · · · 85
THE POSITION IN WALKING · · · · · · 87
   Proper Position · · · · · · · · · 87
   Military Position · · · · · · · · · 88
THE BALANCE STEP · · · · · · · · 89
   Without Gaining Ground · · · · · · · 89
   Gaining Ground · · · · · · · · · 90
WALKING · · · · · · · · · · · 91
   Walking in General · · · · · · · · 91
   General Mechanism of Walking · · · · · 93
   The Slow Walk, or March · · · · · · 94
   The Moderate and the Quick Pace · · · · 96

The Moderate Pace · · · · · · · · · 98
The Quick Pace · · · · · · · · · · 98
Slow Step · · · · · · · · · · · 101
Quick Step · · · · · · · · · · · 101
Double March · · · · · · · · · · 102
Particular Utility of Walking · · · · · · 103
RUNNING AND LEAPING · · · · · · · · 105
EXERCISES OF THE FEET · · · · · · · · 105
Bends in Position · · · · · · · · · 105
Battements in Position · · · · · · · · 108
The Circles, or *Ronds de Jambes* · · · · · 110

PART III

COMBINATIONS OF EXERCISE

DANCING · · · · · · · · · · · · 113
General Remarks · · · · · · · · · 113
General Utility of Dancing · · · · · · · 124
Style · · · · · · · · · · · · 125
Of the Feet, &c. · · · · · · · · · 126
Of the Arms and Hands · · · · · · · 128
Of the Bust · · · · · · · · · · 130
Of the Head · · · · · · · · · · 131
Of the Whole Figure · · · · · · · · 132
Peculiar Manner · · · · · · · · · 133
Continuance · · · · · · · · · · 134
Particular Utility of Dancing · · · · · · 134

PART IV

APPLICATIONS OF EXERCISES TO THE CONDUCT OF LIFE

DEPORTMENT · 139

APPENDIX

GAMES · 153
Le Diable Boiteux · 154
La Grace · 154
Skipping Rope · 154
Shuttlecock and Battledore 155
Bow and Arrow, &c. 155
APPROPRIATION OF EXERCISE · 155
GUIDANCE OF EXERCISES · 163

MEDICAL TESTIMONIALS

Letter from Dr Birkbeck to the author . . . 169
Letter from Dr Copland to the author . . . 171

LIST OF PLATES

Plates

I	Wrong and Right Position in Writing	·	·	20
II	Wrong and Right Position in Drawing	·	·	21
III	Wrong and Right Position in Guitar-Playing			24
IV	Wrong and Right Position in Harp-Playing		·	26
V	Wrong and Right Position in Riding	·	·	27
VI	Wrong and Right Position in Lying in Bed		·	30
VII	The Curved Spine and the Natural one		·	36
VIII	Fundamental and Other Positions	·	·	· 60
IX	Positions in Dancing ·	·	·	·	· 62
X & XI	Extension Motions ·	·	·	·	· 66–67
XII	Exercises with the Rod ·	·	·	·	· 70
XIII & XIV	Exercises with Dumb-Bells	·	·	·	73–74
XV to XXI	Indian Sceptre Exercise ·	·	·	·	77–84
XXII	Walking – The Slow Walk	·	·	·	· 92
XXIII	Walking – The Moderate Pace	·	·	· 95
XXIV	Walking – The Quick Pace ·	·	·	· 97
XXV	Exercises of the Feet – Bends and *Battements* ·	·	·	·	· 106
XXVI	Exercises of the Feet – *Battements* and Circles ·	·	·	·	· 107

XXVII Deportment – The Curtsey · · · · 140

XXVIII Deportment – The Curtsey, &c. · · · 142

XXIX Deportment – Getting into
Carriage, &c. · · · · · · · 150

PECULIARITIES OF THE PRESENT SYSTEM

IT is universally complained that the exercises for ladies at present taught are in many instances frivolous, in other instances severe, in all destitute of system; and the employment of soldiers to teach young ladies to walk, a practice adopted by many parents and heads of seminaries, is generally deprecated.

The military principles of exercise are in most instances excellent; but the stiffness acquired under the practical tuition of sergeants and corporals, is justly observed to be 'adverse to all the principles of grace, and destructive of that buoyant lightness which is so conducive to ease and elegance in the young.'

It is my wish here to combine whatever is really good in the military principles, and in the exercises for ladies as at present taught, to reject what is injurious, to add what seems equally new and necessary, and to present a system suited to the female constitution, nature, and character.

Of the exercises which I here recommend, none accordingly require more strength than the young female possesses, none entail the slightest inconvenience, and all, while they best bestow health, strength, and activity, are calculated to preserve grace and beauty. The whole, I trust, are well suited to the development of the physical faculties in young females, without injury to the perfection of the moral ones.

The introductory views which I give of the structure of the body as connected with exercise – of its functions as affected by exercise; of the constraint to which it is wrongly subjected; of the debility which this causes; of the wrong positions which result from this debility and from the particular pursuits of education when ill directed; of the deformity in which these terminate; of the injury to health and to intellect which accompanies this; and of the particular and special utility of exercises – these views will be acceptable to every parent who desires to know the reasoning by which is guided the education of those who are dearest to him.

The particular exercises, as already said, equally reject whatever is frivolous and whatever is severe, retaining all that contributes to health, strength, beauty of form, and grace of motion.

To obtain the correct position of the figure, the military position of the whole figure,[1] the positions for the feet in dancing, the military extensions for the arms, and the Spanish exercise, are given.

To increase the power and freedom of the arms, the use of dumb-bells, and, which is far more valuable, that of

---

1. The military principles and practices are duly appreciated throughout this work, as those found by the most extensive experience on the most unfavourable subjects, to be upon the whole the best calculated to prevent or remedy every tendency to deformity.

the Indian sceptres, is described – the latter deriving its name from the form of the instrument which ladies employ, instead of the Indian Clubs used by men. A few of the simplest and most elementary of these exercises are now taught to soldiers for the same purpose for which they are here given: all the more graceful ones are here for the first time added for ladies. The latter will be found to be by far the most useful and most beautiful exercises that ever were introduced into physical education; having vast advantages over the dumb-bells in both these respects, and rendering indeed all other exercises for the arms quite useless. *Of these beautiful exercises, both the more simple military ones, and the more advanced and graceful ones now added, are here for the first time described in any work.*

To improve the lower limbs, the position in walking, the balance step, the mechanism of walking in all the paces, and various exercises for the feet, are described; the art of walking well being particularly attended to, *and more accurately described than usual.*

Observations on dancing are subjoined; a series of remarks on deportment, &c. are added; and games of exercise are noticed.

Lastly, the appropriation and guidance of exercises are discussed.

PART I

REASONINGS ON WHICH ARE FOUNDED THE EXERCISES HERE EMPLOYED

OF THE STRUCTURE OF THE BODY AS CONNECTED WITH EXERCISE

OF THE BODY GENERALLY

IN relation to the purpose of exercise, the body may be regarded as composed of many levers, connected with and moveable upon each other in various degrees.

The BONES more especially constitute the levers, upon which all the greater motions depend.

The JOINTS or articulations at once connect these levers, and facilitate their motion.

To form these joints, the ends of the bones are rounded, remarkably smooth, and lubricated with a peculiar liquid; are surrounded by protecting capsules or bags; and are united, laterally or otherwise, by ligaments, which limit the direction of their motions. Between some of their ends exist also moveable cartilages, by which their motions are extended, and all shocks which pass through them are diminished.

The MUSCLES, generally disposed in pairs on each side of the body, are the moving powers.

These bundles of muscular fibres form the layers and masses of flesh which lie between the skin and the various bones, which cover the neck, the back, the sides, the pelvis or haunches and hips, and which principally give shape to the limbs. Almost every muscle is fixed to two different bones by its extremities; and its middle in general passes more loosely over one or more joints which it is destined to move.

Of the peculiar mechanism of muscular motion, it is enough here to say, that these muscles receive nerves which communicate with the lesser brain (the cerebel or organ of the will); and when that organ wills a movement, it, through these nerves, excites those muscles which are to be the means of the particular operation to shorten and swell up. Now, as the muscles cannot bring their fixed extremities nearer to each other without also bringing, along with these, the bones to which they are attached, the intermediate joint or joints are bent, and motion takes place in the limb, or throughout the body.

Such is the general mechanism of all our greater motions.

OF THE VERTEBRAL COLUMN IN PARTICULAR

One of the most important portions of this locomotive fabric is the vertebral column, spinal column, or backbone, as it is commonly called.

The backbone is a pillar composed of twenty-four short

bones, called vertebrae, having somewhat cylindrical bodies before, a bony ring in the middle, an irregular projection on each side, and another altogether behind. These are placed one upon another, the smaller being always upper-most; and they extend from the large bones that support the body, when sitting, to the lowest part of the head.

These small bones or vertebrae are connected togeth-er by the whole of the flat upper and under surfaces of their bodies, a thick cartilage being interposed between every two; and they are also connected by the apposition of certain lateral projections or processes. They are main-tained in their relative position by means of small bundles of strong and elastic ligamentous fibres, attached firmly to the margins of their bodies, and to the projections of every two bones.

The position of the backbone or spinal column, thus formed and connected, is, in all its lateral relations to the plane on which we stand, perfectly perpendicular; but it is naturally curved anteriorly and posteriorly.

While, by the cartilaginous connexion of the bodies of the vertebrae, and by the disposition of some parts of the projections that have been mentioned, joints are formed, and provision is made for the column being bent in every direction, other projections allow certain muscles at once to take firm hold, and greatly to increase their purchase in actually bending the spinal column.

The moving power of the vertebral column is composed of these muscles. Being chiefly attached to the sides and back of each vertebra, they form two considerable masses of fleshy fibres placed one on each side of the ridge in the middle of the back.

These masses exert such balancing power over every separate bone or vertebra in relation to or upon that placed immediately beneath it, as to keep the whole pile at rest and upright, in regard to its lateral aspect. They bend it also both laterally and backward. It is chiefly by other muscles on the fore part of the body that it is bended forwards. By the whole, it may be bent in any requisite direction within certain limits; and, after performing its various inflexions, it is, by means of its elastic ligaments and other muscles, enabled to regain the vertical position.

Thus each of the four-and-twenty vertebrae, or small bones of the spinal column, is a lever, whose support or fulcrum is the upper surface of the somewhat larger vertebra upon which it rests.

IMPORTANT CIRCUMSTANCES TO BE NOTED

Having very briefly described this column, it is here especially necessary to observe, that the bones of adults owe their solidity to an earthy material, called phosphate of lime; but that the bones of infants contain very little of this matter, and are, accordingly, very soft and flexible. In proportion, however, as more earthy matter is added, the bones of children become harder and less flexible; and this hardening increases till the prime of life, when no trace of the soft part, or cartilage, on or in which the bony matter was deposited, can be observed. The progress of this hardening of the bones may, by various causes, be accelerated or retarded. This, obviously, is important in relation to the constrained positions to which girls are subjected.

It is equally worthy of observation that, in youth, all the bones are formed in various distinct pieces, and that these pieces long continue very imperfectly connected. Thus every long bone consists of three separate pieces during early youth, and these do not become perfectly consolidated till the age of sixteen, eighteen, or later. This also is important in relation to the constrained positions to which girls are subjected.

It is perhaps still more worthy of observation, that not only do these causes of flexibility exist in the bones in general, but that, in relation to the vertebral column, or backbone, the substance interposed between every two vertebrae – the intervertebral substance – is liable, by long-continued pressure or extension, to be permanently altered in thickness at any part, and thereby to alter also the direction of the vertebral column. This is, perhaps, still more important in relation to the constrained positions to which girls are subjected.

It is most worthy of observation, that throughout the centre of this flexible spinal column exists a somewhat three-sided tube, for the purpose of containing the portion of the nervous system, improperly denominated the spinal marrow, a nervous or brainy production, on which the sensation and motion of the body and limbs depend, and which is connected superiorly with the greater brain before, and the lesser behind. This is of the very greatest importance in relation to the constrained positions to which girls are subjected.

———————

OF THE FUNCTIONS OF THE BODY AS AFFECTED BY EXERCISE

THE movements of the body are of two kinds.

The first take place without consciousness or any act of the will. They consist of the exercise of the vital functions for the preservation and support of life; as of the stomach, intestines, heart, &c. and also of the exercise of all the muscles when they act involuntarily.

The second are the movements performed consciously and voluntarily, when we put in action any muscle for a particular purpose. It is these last which constitute exercise.

By exercise, the power of the muscular fibres is increased.

When a limb is moved, the muscles which are actuated swell by the more frequent and copious flow of blood into them, and heat is developed. If the motion be long continued, the limb grows stiff; a sensation of lassitude is felt; and a difficulty of further contraction is the result. If the motion were violent, and the blood were called in excess into the limb, inflammation might arise.

If, on the contrary, after intervals of repose, we perform the same motions, and many times repeat this, we observe an increase of bulk and energy in the part, in consequence of the more active conversion of nutritious matters into its substance, and also a perfection of action which was not previously enjoyed.

Hence, in labouring men, the limbs employed in their occupation are larger in proportion than the rest: this is the case with the arms of smiths, bakers, boxers, wrestlers, &c. and the legs of porters, couriers, dancers, &c.

This increase of size has nothing to do with fatness: on the contrary, exercise tends to make the body lean. Labouring men, hunters, and soldiers, are not fat; but their flesh is firm and strong, because the habit of exercise has conferred these qualities on their muscles.

This effect is still more evident amongst animals.

Those cooped up where they cannot sufficiently employ their muscles, have the flesh delicate, tender, white and fat, and are without strength enough to escape from their destroyer. The flesh of wild fowls, on the contrary, is firm, hard, dark coloured, and lean – proofs of strength and vigour.

Generally speaking, the effect of active exercises on any part, or any animal, is greater the more it is in motion.

The person, however, who is constantly employed in muscular exercises never acquires great strength. If continued exercises are also violent, what is gained does not make up for what is lost, and he wastes quickly.

If, on the contrary, exercise and repose are alternate, it favours nutrition and the development of muscular power.

The person, then, who acquires the greatest strength is he who practises muscular exercises which require great force, but who follows them up by sufficient intervals of repose.

To have an idea of the extensive effects of exercise on the rest of the organization, it is enough to observe that the locomotive muscles and their levers, the bones, form a mass much larger and heavier than all the other organs, and that their actions also are by far the largest and most powerful. It is thence evident how vast must be the influence of the repeated and continued action of such organs on the rest of the economy.

When the body is in a state of repose, the interior functions are, indeed, in exercise; but, as the organs which execute them do not receive any impulse or excitement from without, their action is slow and feeble. Not only the muscles themselves lose their suppleness and energy; the whole organization is enfeebled; and, if the state of repose continue, the strongest man will ultimately become weak and indisposed.

On the contrary, under the influence of exercise, the interior functions increase in activity and power.

It has been observed that the cerebel, or little brain, by means of the nerves acting upon the muscles, excites them to produce motion: it may now be added that the heart gives to the muscles a similar excitement, or rather, the means of acting by pouring into them the blood; because, if we were to intercept the blood which is sent to them by that organ, they would soon be unable to contract, and their active power would finally cease.

Thus the nervous system and the system of the blood-vessels are evidently the two principal causes which determine the muscular contractions.

As, however, everything is united and dependant in the economy of animal life, the muscles cannot be put in action or be exercised without reacting on the brain by means of other nerves, and on the heart by means of the returning vessels or veins. Thus the heart and brain, being again more stimulated, return an additional stimulus to the muscles themselves, and to all the organs.

In this way, the contractions of the muscles produce a

general excitement, making all the organs partake of their activity. It is thus that everyone must have observed, after active exercise, those effects (the very causes of which we are now explaining) namely, palpitation of the heart, high pulse, heat, redness of the skin, perspiration, &c.

If we now wish, for example's sake, to apply these simple physiological principles to explain the influence of exercise upon digestion, we can understand how the organs whose duty it is to perform this vital function, increase, by exercise, in strength and power. If the stomach be empty, exercise accordingly creates or increases the appetite, and ensures a more speedy, easy, and perfect, digestion. It must, however, be observed that violent exercise too long continued exhausts the common energy of all the organs, and consequently troubles and disorders the movements of the stomach, and thus injures the digestion.

As to the circulation, it has already been seen that exercise accelerates the palpitations of the heart and the action of the blood-vessels. The same thing occurs with respiration, which becomes quick in proportion to the force and activity of our external motions.

It is, however, in its effect upon the nourishment and material composition of the body, that it is most interesting, in relation to the present views, to notice the consequence of exercise. It is especially in contributing to this function that exercise spreads heat and vital energy equally over the body, and maintains an equilibrium among all the functions.

Even the sensations receive from action new excitement. We know that, after long repose, the intellect becomes dull, and that by the effect of exercise, not so great as to fatigue, perceptions of some kinds arise more freely, and the intellectual faculties are reanimated.

Sleep, on the contrary, placing the brain in an inactive state, it follows that its too frequent repetition, and especially its excessive prolongation, must enervate that organ. Thus, too much sleep not only benumbs the brain, it also directly debilitates it.

It appears, however, that active muscular exercises leave those particular organs of the brain which have reference to moral qualities and intellectual faculties in a state of repose. The action of the brain during exercise seems limited to those of its organs which direct the movements.

The local effects of active exercises, or those that take place in the members in action, when these exercises are carried too far, are, as has been said, inflammation of the muscles, rheumatism, &c.

The general effects of too great indulgence in muscular exercises, are the exhaustion of the cerebral and spinal nervous system, and proportionally of all the organs depending thereon.

If exercise be indulged in too much, but not so constantly, it makes individuals appear prematurely old.

This last is an important consideration to those for whom this work is written. The error they commit, however, is not likely to be of this, but the opposite kind, which is more surely and immediately fatal to health and beauty.

———————

OF THE CONSTRAINT TO WHICH THE
BODY IS WRONGLY SUBJECTED

THE excessive, or too long continued, action of locomotive organs, is not so frequently injurious to them in women, as is the state of inactivity, arising from constraint, by which their structure is often wasted and their capability of action lost.

I agree with Dr Duffin that 'the state of deficiency in the consolidation of the bodies of the vertebrae results, in many instances, from the present enfeebling system of conducting female education,' and that stays, adding constraint to enfeeblement, 'prove doubly injurious if used before the body has acquired its full growth, because, at that period especially, the body is capable of being moulded into any shape the fashion of the time may consider most becoming,' a circumstance which the Doctor illustrates by a striking diagram, for which I refer the reader to his excellent work.[1]

I dissent, however, from the Doctor in his thinking that 'a moderate and equable degree of compression, given to muscles much called into exercise, so that it does not unduly interfere with their power of contraction, is undoubtedly beneficial.'

There is, I will venture to assert, no 'compression of muscles' that does not 'interfere with their power of contraction,' or that is not injurious exactly in proportion to its 'degree'; and the more muscles are 'called into action,'

1. A somewhat similar drawing is given by the celebrated physician Soemmering; but I have not seen it.

the more injurious must such 'compression' always be! This mistake arises from the utility, real or supposed, of belts around the loins; but such utility, if it exists, depends on their supporting the internal abdominal organs, not on their 'compression of muscles'.

The Doctor's views on this subject, however, are generally much bolder than those of his predecessors, and this, I believe, is the only faulty concession he makes to popular opinion. Hence it is with great truth that, speaking practically, the Doctor says 'Remove the constraint of dress, and the young lady instantly complains of weakness in her back – of inability to support herself erect.'[2]

To the constraint of dress, is added the absence, I may almost say the impossibility, of exercise.

The only exercises, indeed, to which, in their hours of relaxation, young ladies have access, are in general only a few insignificant games, or amusements extremely limited, from the nature of the space afforded for the purposes of exercise. Even these are in general carefully prohibited as soon as the pupils enter into them with ardour, and perhaps properly so; for exercise indulged in without any regulation might produce real inconveniences, which a system composed of select exercises, suited to the age and strength of the pupil, does not produce.

––––––––––

2. In speaking thus freely of this able writer and practitioner, who is doing far more than any other to correct the barbarous practices in institutions for female education, I give the best proof of perfect impartiality.

OF THE DEBILITY WHICH IS
CAUSED BY CONSTRAINT

IT has been already said that continued repose of a member decreases nutrition in it, and subjects it to waste: the irritability caused by movement not taking place, the flow of the blood which it caused ceases also.

To decrease of nutrition, appears to be added a weakening of the function from want of use: the member having been for some time in a state of repose, has no longer similar power.

The proofs of this are innumerable; being afforded by all the acts of our lives in which habit is more or less irregular. We feel that they are less perfectly repeated after intervals of cessation.

If this repose endure for a long time, movement of the limb becomes almost impossible.

It would appear also that, with the enfeebling of the muscles and the diminution of the calibre of their vessels, occurs also a defect in the exhalation of the membranes of the joints or articulations.

When to this is added that pressure which produces absorption and waste of the supporting muscles, the organic injury is at its height – the means of adequate support are gone. A medical friend mentions to me an instance, which he himself witnessed, of several of the muscles of the neck being partially divided by the long continued use of a tight necklace.

Hence persons who have long been accustomed to the support of tight stays find it almost impossible to lay them aside, because their sudden discontinuance induces the most distressing feeling of the weakness which constraint has produced.

Unhappily, the means almost always employed to compensate for this persevering destruction of natural power, is increased use of its causes.

The final consequence of this is stated by Portal, who says, 'Persons adopting such means, are sure to become distorted whenever the artificial props are removed.'

————

OF THE WRONG POSITIONS WHICH RESULT FROM DEBILITY, AND FROM THE EMPLOYMENT, IN THE PARTICULAR PURSUITS OF EDUCATION, OR THE COMMON ACTS OF LIFE, OF MUSCLES UNFAVOURABLY SITUATED

Now, the use of stays and other restraints, as well as sedentary habits, causing, in the manner just described, debility of many of the muscles, naturally induces the use, in the particular pursuits of education or the common acts of life, of other muscles, of which the power is less impaired, but which are less favourably situated for the purpose in view.

This is the great cause of wrong positions of the figure, and all their fatal consequences.

The following are a few of the most remarkable of the wrong positions resulting from debility or from the improper employment of the muscles in such cases. All of them have been more or less noticed by writers on deformity, except perhaps that connected with the guitar and the corrective means it may afford, the peculiar effects of riding on horseback, and the general truth as to one-sidedness to which most of them tend.

IN STANDING

Boys compelled to stand during a long lesson relieve the muscles that maintain the body erect, by balancing themselves on one leg, which is generally the left, in order that the more active right may be free. This throws out the hip, hollows the body, and depresses the shoulder of the side on which they stand. If this be the left, it raises the right shoulder.

Girls, during the same act, relieve themselves by passing one hand round the back, so as to support it, and they thereby draw down the opposite elbow, and consequently the opposite shoulder.

IN SITTING

By sitting always on the same side of the fire or window, persons lean to one side, and thereby depress the shoulder of that side, and raise the opposite one.

Girls, in sitting, contract a habit of balancing the body upon one hip, and of throwing on it the weight of all the parts above it, by drawing the spine to that side, and leaning the head and neck to the other. This raises relatively the shoulder of the side on which they rest, as is seen when they stand erect and carefully retain the same position of the trunk.

PLATE I

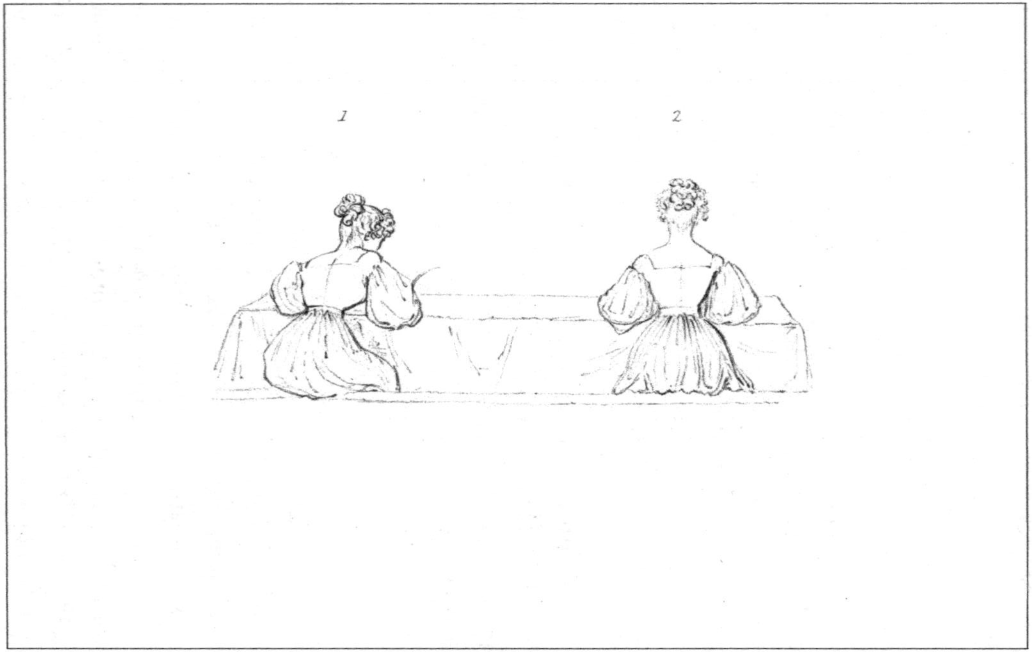

WRONG AND RIGHT POSITION IN WRITING

PLATE II

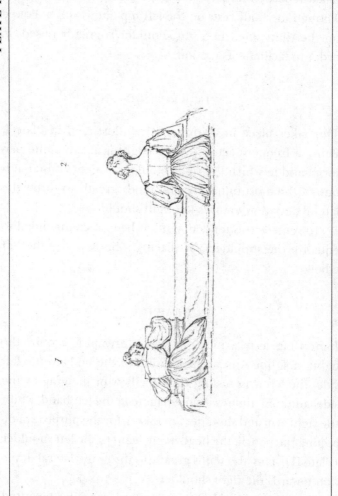

WRONG AND RIGHT POSITION IN DRAWING

A deviation from this circumstance (of the shoulder of the side on which they rest being raised in sitting) takes place in occupations which engage the right hand and arm. Though the body rests on the left hip and is still hollowed on the right side, the right shoulder is greatly raised, in order to facilitate its motion.

IN WRITING

This takes place in writing, and is illustrated in Plate I. Being a frequent act, which the right arm can alone perform, and in which the right shoulder is always raised, it is one of the most injurious, and tends greatly to throw the lateral deviation towards the right shoulder.

To remedy this tendency, it has been recommended to equalize the shoulders, by placing a book under the left elbow.

IN DRAWING

In drawing, as in writing, both sexes are apt to acquire the habit of sitting with an inclination of the body to the left side, the left arm resting on the elbow or hanging by the side, and sometimes with the palette in the left hand, whilst the right arm and shoulder are raised, for the purpose of directing the pencil, the head being leant to the left shoulder (Plate II). This also tends greatly to throw the lateral deviation towards the right shoulder.

The able artist, Mr Frank Howard, who has favoured me by making the Drawings for this work, and whose creative mind and ready hand have in these, as in many other matters, no rival with which I am acquainted, obliges me also by the following valuable observations on the false position in drawing.

On the position in drawing, I would only add to your description of the improper one, that there is a tendency to throw all the weight on the left elbow, for the purpose of having greater liberty with the right arm; and that the evil of this is increased by the height of the desk or table on which the drawing is placed. A habit is thus contracted of leaning over the drawing, and resting the chest against the edge of the table, which is productive of contraction, of vital derangements, and at the same time of a cramped manner of drawing, sufficiently objectionable in itself.

The proper position, when sitting, is to have the drawing considerably lower than the waist, and to sit erect without throwing any weight on the left hip, elbow, or hand. The drawing can be seen better, the whole of it being visible at one glance; and much greater freedom in the style must result from the removal of the real constraint of the right arm.

In fact, the object for which so much is sacrificed in the false position, is gained in the true one, without any sacrifice at all. It is admitted that in the false position, there is not so much liberty for the hand to disobey the eye – it cannot go so far or so fast in an erroneous direction; but this mode of controlling the hand is quite a delusion, as in the true position it will have much greater scope to obey the mind, which, after all, is the only true source whence capability of drawing is derived.

PLATE III

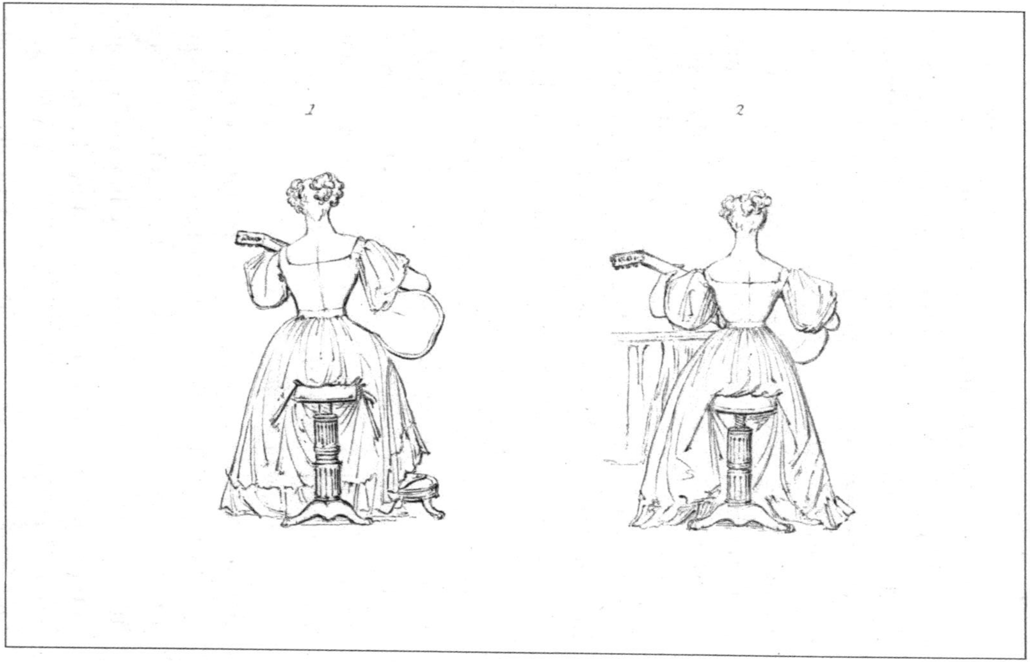

WRONG AND RIGHT POSITION IN GUITAR-PLAYING

The advantages, therefore, of commencing drawing in the true position are twofold; first, with regard to the attainment of the art, and, secondly, with regard to the preservation of health and of beauty of figure.

IN GUITAR-PLAYING

In playing on the guitar, in some instances, the right knee is elevated to support the instrument, and the right shoulder is slightly raised. This is avoided by the far preferable position of Fernando Sor (Plate III). The practice alluded to, therefore, tends further to throw the lateral deviation towards the right shoulder.

More frequently, perhaps, the guitar is rested in the lap, the left foot is placed on a stool, and the left shoulder is raised. This of course tends to throw the deviation in that direction.

The present is the proper place to observe that, for a lady who also plays on the harp, or is engaged much in any other pursuit which tends to raise the right shoulder, the last mode of playing on the guitar, which raises the left shoulder, is preferable, as counteracting the opposite tendency of the other pursuit.

On this observation as to these two instruments, may be founded a general rule as to finding similar compensations in all.

Unfortunately, however, these pursuits are in general solitary; and their peculiar tendency to the right or to the left, is unchecked by any other countervailing circumstance. Nay, when one is a principal and predominating occupation, there always exists a strong tendency to assume

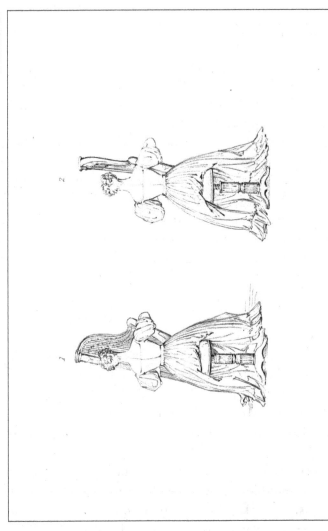

PLATE IV

WRONG AND RIGHT POSITION IN HARP-PLAYING

PLATE V

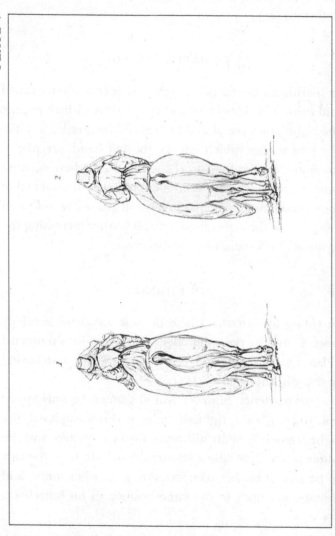

WRONG AND RIGHT POSITION IN RIDING

the same attitude and position in every other action of life. Hence an insensibly growing, and at last irremediable, deformity.

IN HARP-PLAYING

In playing on the harp, the right shoulder is at once raised and thrown back, because the treble strings, which engage the right hand, are placed higher and further back; while the bass strings, which engage the left hand, are placed lower and further forward (Plate IV). Here, then, occurs a twist of the body which cannot fail of being detrimental to those who have not attained their full growth, as well as an elevation of the right shoulder, still further increasing the tendency to deviation in that direction.

IN RIDING

In riding on horseback, the body is somewhat similarly twisted, and the right shoulder is apt to be thrown upward (Plate V), increasing apparently the tendency to deviation in that direction.[3]

This tendency, however, will in general be only apparent; for, while the right shoulder is thrown upward, the right haunch is often still more thrown upward, and the whole of the right side is shortened; so that, were the lady to be placed on her feet, extending only her limbs, and holding her body in the same position as on horseback,

3. In Figure 1, the inclination is rather too much. *In general,* it is much less.

with the right side contracted, the right shoulder would in reality be depressed, and the tendency to deviation would be to the left side.

Thus, riding on horseback might also perhaps be employed as counteracting the far more general tendency to raise the right shoulder, which is produced by the more frequent and longer continued acts of writing, drawing, &c., and by the perpetual employment of the right hand in all the acts of common life, which compel the greater or lesser liberation of the shoulder from the corset or stays, its increased development, and the almost universal tendency to right-sided deviation and deformity.

I feel, however, the greatest objection to riding on horseback as an exercise for ladies, on other accounts; namely, the twist which it gives to the whole body; the elevation which it produces of one of the shoulders; the immense increase which it causes in the waist by incessantly employing and developing the large muscles of the sides, in order to secure the rider's balance (and this too in a nation where slenderwaistedness is beauty!); the enfeeblement and deformity which it causes in the thighs, legs, and feet;[4] the coarseness of voice, which is always caused by conversing in a loud tone with a riding companion; the increased exposure to weather, which is so unfavourable to the complexion; the early improper irritation and subsequent debility which it produces;[5] the unnatural consolidation of the bones of the

4. See the regiments of Guards, in which I never could discover an old trooper who had two legs alike!

5. The history of the Cossack women, who are much on horseback, illustrates this.

PLATE VI

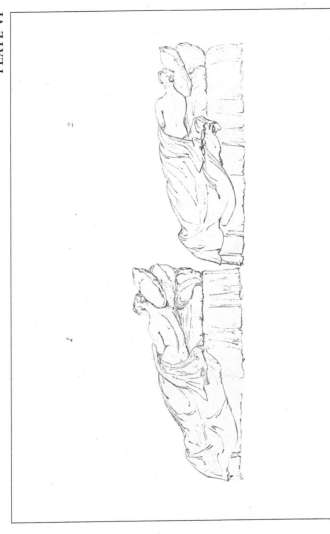

WRONG AND RIGHT POSITION IN LYING IN BED

lower part of the body, ensuring a dangerous and frightful impediment to future functions which need not here be dwelt on; in short, its altogether masculine and unwomanly character.

IN LYING IN BED

In sleeping on a feather-bed, with high pillows, the body is not only enervated, but, as we generally lie on the right side, the right shoulder is again raised, and the tendency to deviation in that direction still further increased.

The spine is also twisted, and the neck turned awry (Plate VI).

When two children sleep in one bed, they seldom fail, unless they change sides, to contract a habit of lying always on the same side of the body; and when this is practised every night during several years, it can scarcely fail to produce deformity.

———————

Thus, as the most frequent curvature of the spine is lateral, its causes are also lateral; and those are egregiously mistaken who imagine that its cause is ever perpendicular. They fail to observe that, when lateral curvature arises, even from some fault in a foot, it is solely because its influence is laterally applied, through the oblique neck of the thigh-bone, that it can have the slightest effect on the spinal column. Considered both in its relation to surgery and to my present subject – exercise – this is a simple, clear and important principle, now enunciated, I believe, for the first time.

Thus also the tendency of the greater number of the acts I have described, and especially of the frequent and long-continued act of writing, the similarly continued act of drawing, and the long enduring state of sleep, is added to that of all the acts of common life, in producing deviation and deformity, primarily and fundamentally, towards the right shoulder; and it is for these reasons that deviations to that side so greatly exceed those in the opposite direction.

OF THE DEFORMITY IN WHICH WRONG POSITIONS TERMINATE

THE INJURY THUS DONE TO THE LOCOMOTIVE ORGANS AND FUNCTIONS, OR THOSE ON WHICH GENERAL MOTION DEPENDS

As this matter is well described by Dr Duffin, I owe to him the immediately following observations, on which I have made few and slight alterations.

It has been already shown that the intervertebral substance holds together the two vertebrae or bones of the spine between which it is interposed; and, though it firmly adheres to the opposed surfaces of both, and prevents their loose or free action, it yet permits a most extensive motion of the whole column of bones, taken conjointly, in consequence of the great elastic power of which it is possessed.

To whichever side the body inclines, the intervertebral substance readily yields; and, when the weight of the body and the force of muscular contraction have ceased to bend the spine to any particular side, it returns in a moment to its proper position, by a powerful resilience of this substance, and the aid of antagonist muscles.

Now, even in a healthy and vigorous individual, an unequal action of the originally symmetrical masses of muscle, which have already been described as situated laterally and posteriorly to the spinal column, if this action be frequent, excessive, or protracted, may evidently impart an unsymmetrical form to the bones which they powerfully and perpetually influence; and if so, how much more easily would the same organs, acting unequally, induce deformity in the delicate female who is subject to perpetual constraint, who is consequently enfeebled, and to whom wrong position has become habitual!

In a healthy woman, a double curvature of the spine may be brought on by the habit of always nursing her child on her left arm. Clerks and other sedentary persons, frequently contract the lateral, or twisted curvature. Ploughmen have the right shoulder much higher than the left. Sailors have generally the spine bent forward.

> It is notorious that artisans, generally, contract some bend or twist in their backbone or limbs, so characteristic as to enable a practised eye easily to judge of their respective pursuits, without any other information than what is derived from their appearance.

In short,

> any undue inclination to either side during life, if frequent, constant, or protracted, will cause a certain diminution in the thickness of this (the intervertebral) substance on the side to which the body inclines,

accompanied by a proportionate rising of the same on the opposite side; and will, in the course of time, produce permanent distortion of the whole column of bones – the result of the compression, and consequent absorption of the intervertebral substance.

This effect will be more easily produced during childhood, when the bones are in a state of growth, the ligaments more yielding, and the intervertebral substance peculiarly soft.

If, owing to constraint, want of exercise, &c.

a due supply of blood be not afforded to the bones of the spine, they will be so much nearer to the state of cartilage than they ought to be; and will consequently yield more readily to the operation of any undue or partial pressure.

In young persons subject to the causes already described,

the bones of the spine never become firm, yield easily to the superincumbent weight, aided perhaps by the force of the muscles; and thus, being disposed to grow unequally, impart to the spine a lateral inclination of longer or shorter continuance.

The spine thus deviates from its natural direction, slightly at first, but, finally, to such an extent as to make it betray its want of symmetry, even to the most indifferent observer.

This deformity

very rarely manifests itself before the child has attained the seventh or eighth year of age. From this period to the sixteenth or eighteenth year, the highest degree of excitability of the nervous system exists.

There are few mothers who are not familiar with one of the first characteristics of this affliction – a projecting, high, and distorted shoulder.

On a more careful examination, it is found that the central groove of the back deviates from a straight line; that there is a greater distance between a given point of the original perpendicular spinal line and the top of the elevated shoulder bone, than between the same point and the corresponding top of the opposite side. As the deformity advances, the gait of the young person becomes awkward and shuffling; her clothes cannot be made to fit well upon her; they appear to be drawn to one side, generally the right. The sash encircling her waist is observed to dip in the same direction, while the right breast presents a more than ordinary fullness, and the corresponding collarbone displays a proportionate elevation. In short, the child is deformed. Her backbone is distorted.

In proportion as the inclination takes place in the upper part of the back, between the shoulders, nature, in order to counterbalance the evil, and preserve the equilibrium of the body, calls into action the muscles of the lower part of the spine on the opposite side; so that, in confirmed cases, a double curvature is produced.

As the infirmity advances, a similar counterpoising power is exerted by the muscles of the spine attached to the vertebrae of the neck, and a third or upper curve is then formed, so that the spine presents a serpentine appearance, inclining to each side alternately.

PLATE VII

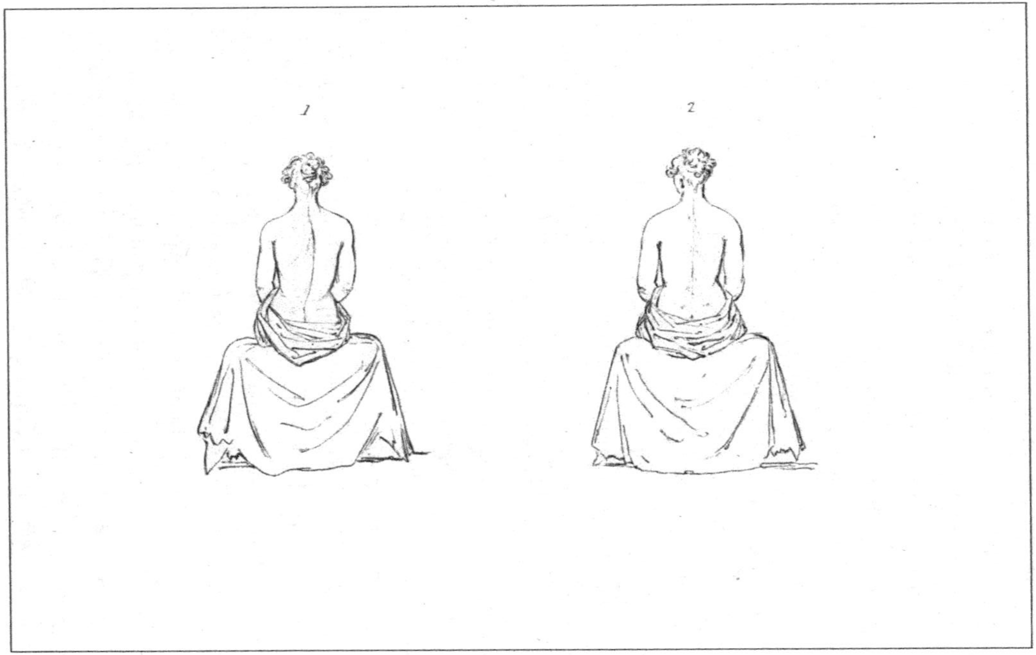

THE CURVED SPINE AND THE NATURAL ONE

The ribs, in consequence of the alteration in the course of the spine, aided by a continuance of the same debilitating causes, soon partake of the extending change that is going on, and, deviating from their true direction, contract and deform the chest.

Finally, the basin or pelvis, on which the spine rests, becoming involved, produces an inequality in the size of the hips, the contrary of that which obtains in the shoulder, and causes the body, when viewed from behind, to appear as if twisted on itself. [See Plate VII, where this is contrasted with the natural and beautiful form.]

The longer the deformity exists, unless the causes whence it proceeds be discontinued, the more conspicuous it is sure to become.

Pinaeus, who flourished towards the close of the sixteenth century, asserts (so common was it at that period) 'that of fifty females of the higher or more civilized ranks of society, scarcely two could be found who had not the right shoulder higher, and more projecting, than the left,' an assertion which, but slightly modified, may, with considerable truth, be applied to young women of a corresponding class in modern times.

The Doctor might, I believe, with truth, have said that, in later times and in the great capitals, Pinaeus' estimate would be under, rather than over the truth.

During childhood, backboards, steel stays, constrained positions of the body, concealed pressure, and similar expedients, are resorted to with a view to force in, or

bind down, the high and projecting shoulder, errone-
ously supposed to be alone in fault. This treatment, it
need hardly be observed, is almost invariably productive of an aggravation of the mischief it is designed to
remedy, as well as injurious to the form of the chest.

If the shoulders be braced by means of straps to a
plate of iron placed on the back, it is evident that the
action of the muscles, with which nature has endowed
the body for the express purpose of holding the
shoulders in a graceful position, will be superseded,
and will, from want of due use, become proportionately
incapable of performing their wonted office when the
strap is removed.

Artifices of dress being now substituted for mechanical contrivances, the manipulations of the waiting-maid
supply the place of well-directed medical and surgical
skill; or, in more pointed cases, the machinist is resorted
to, who not unfrequently increases the deformity he
undertakes to cure.

Machines, of every description, for the prevention
of deformity, or for the cure of bad habits, should be
avoided: they are at best very inefficient substitutes for
the means provided by nature. In young persons, in
whom we may wish to correct round shoulders, or a
habit of stooping, we can obtain our object, and at the
same time improve the general health and strength,
more by the superintendence of their exercises and
amusements, so as to make a moderate demand for
muscular exertion on particular parts of the body,
than by the use of backboards, collars, or any kind of
mechanical contrivance.

I have, on the subject of this section, quoted Dr Duffin as the best medical describer of this particular but almost universal deformity, and I call him so from no personal intimacy or possibility of interest, for I have seen him but a few times, and that only on the subject of his work.

On this point, I have only to add that Riolan, chief physician to Mary de' Medici, observed that most of the women of his time had the right shoulder larger than the left; and that Winslow first showed that, by the pressure of stays, the lower ribs also were depressed, and their cartilaginous portions unnaturally bent.

THE INJURY THUS DONE TO THE VITAL ORGANS AND FUNCTIONS, OR THOSE ON WHICH LIFE DEPENDS

It is well known that the constraints of dress impede the functions of the digestive organs, and lay the foundation of many diseases.

It is equally known that such constraints produce the worst effects on the function of respiration, and consequently on that of circulation generally.

It is not less known, that such constraints, acting on the cellular tissue around the bosom, are not only injurious to the beauty of its form, but expose it to future diseases of the most dangerous kind.

In the same manner, want of exercise prevents all the organs from acquiring that firmness of structure which renders their movements more effective and useful.

As, moreover, active exercise, which brings into action a number of muscles, does not confine its effects to the parts in motion, but influences also the great vital organs contained in the trunk of the body; so does repose of all the muscles influence, in an opposite manner, all the same organs of life.

Want of exercise prevents the liquids from experiencing that transpression which perfects them, by passing frequently through various vessels and filters. Stagnating from want of action on the part of the solids, they spontaneously alter; their composition is deranged; the elements which form them either separate or produce new combinations.

It would indeed appear, that from want of exercise, every vital function decreases in energy, except, in some persons, the oily secretion.

'It is,' says Cabanis, a high authority, here quoted for those less able to observe and reason, 'it is for the most part only the want of bodily movement and respiration in the open air, and some other errors in regimen, food, clothing, &c., which render young women so often ailing, which retard, or derange, or prevent some of their *essential* functions, and which make of them deplorable victims at the age of nubility and of happiness.'

While I am writing this, Sir Anthony Carlisle, who is one of the last, if I mistake not, of the favourite disciples of John Hunter, that remains to us, and who, like that illustrious man, has ever sought to ennoble his profession, by founding all its practice on the great truths of physical science, states to me an important fact, which may with far more propriety be stated by one so profoundly experienced and so justly distinguished, than it can be by me: namely, that the causes which I have here described 'lead especially to an excess of all those bodily infirmities and deformities which, in young women of rank and affluence, destroy their ability to extend their families, and cause the heirship to titles and fortunes to be in general so soon extinguished.'

Those with whom neither reasoning nor these supreme authorities prevail, are reckless of all consequences to the welfare and happiness of their children.

THE INJURY THUS DONE TO THE MENTAL ORGANS AND FUNCTIONS, OR THOSE ON WHICH THOUGHT DEPENDS

The physical constraint to which young women are subjected, is necessarily attended by a mental constraint, which is absurdly mistaken for the means of education. It is indeed for the sake of this education (wretched as it is!) that much of this constraint is endured.

By the word education is meant, not the attention bestowed upon developing the physical and moral faculties, but simply the precocious acquirement of a little fancy needlework, a little French, a little Italian, a little singing, a little dancing, &c.; and this being acquired, the happy parents regard their daughter not as a puppet, mentally as well as bodily enfeebled, but as a model of perfection.

If during the ill-timed struggle to attain this, the young lady's physical constitution has been unable to unfold itself, and she remains weak, pale and nervous, this is imputed to original constitution; and the ruin of strength and health is thus compensated for by the most slight and superficial acquirements.

They forget that, as observed by Dr Duffin, 'in the philosophy of education, doubling the power does not always double the effect. The second hour of study is seldom half so good as the first; the third is much worse than the second ... Experience teaches us, besides, that nothing would be lost by the intervention of amusement, but that an actual accession would be made to the acuteness of the individual.'

They forget that those to whom the education of woman is entrusted ought to know something of her temperament in general, and of her mind in particular.

Anthropologists have observed that the temperament of woman is that of infancy, and that it is marked by weakness and sensibility.

The weakness of woman arises from the extreme tenderness of the fibres of which the muscles are composed, the greater quantity of the cellular tissue which unites them, and the abundance of the juices which moisten them.

This delicacy seems to be naturally accompanied by an openness to impressions, and a sensibility which is lively and easily excited; for when the weakness of woman is increased by any circumstance, the delicacy and susceptibility of the organs become greater, and the sensibility increases to a malady.

Thus is woman far more sensible than man. As, moreover, all the parts and tissues of which woman is formed are finer, more delicate, and more supple, this smallness induces agility; for it is a rule almost without exception, that the smaller animals are, of their particular kind, the more rapid and multiplied are their movements.

Thus is woman, by nature, far more inclined than man to movement, however slight its description.

Indeed, muscular movement and the development of

sensibility arise from a common principle, nervous action, which must be equally employed in both these phenomena.

Now, as exercise strengthens the body, it is easy to conceive that repose must accumulate sensibility; and that unless they alternate with each other, either the one or the other is generated in excess.

Accordingly, in leaving unemployed a considerable part of the muscular fibres, repose enfeebles them directly, and it permits the forces which should actuate them in muscular motion, to follow the central tendency which carries them towards the nervous system.

By this means, all the functions more directly dependent on sensibility acquire great predominance over those which are, properly speaking, only series of physical movements.

Hence, nothing so much foments the passions as solitude and inaction. Hence, the greater number of the affections of girls arise, as de Sévigné says, '*d'avoir toujours le cul sur selle*'.

All the ills, indeed, which afflict the luxurious women of our great cities are a consequence of this error. Lounging on soft couches, protected from cold, heat, atmosphere and light, they are afraid of everything, shun everything, and suffer as much as the unsheltered wretch.

We every day see that if sensibility acquire that influence, which in females of a certain class, the inaction of the muscles and the development of the passions cause it to usurp, the vital powers soon fail in the regularity of their action, and the mental powers become perverted, and in their aberrations, produce nervous diseases.

Hence, then, spring all those convulsive maladies which are much more frequent in feeble and delicate women than in others. They are, indeed, the natural punishment of a life passed in luxury and indolence.

In woman, there is nothing, not even aberration of intellect, erotic and religious insanity, which is not ascribable to the cause now described. All her good and all her bad qualities are the consequences of her weakness and sensibility.

OF THE PARTICULAR AND SPECIAL UTILITY OF EXERCISES

I HAVE stated that the effect of exercise is, by frequent contraction of the fibres, to brace the muscles and render them stronger, and generally to give more strength to the organs.

Nothing evidently can be more suitable to the organization of woman. Her tissues are soft and flexible; exercise renders them more firm and resisting: her fibres are thin and weak; exercise increases their size and strength: they are moistened with oils and juices; exercise diminishes the superabundant humidity.

In regard to strength in general, it may be observed that, in the present state of society, we have less need of it than the people of ancient times. Muscular strength is a kind of superiority no longer in such favour, and the aim of gymnastics is consequently nothing more than to endow the body with all the strength, vigour and activity, compatible with health, without injury to the development of the intellectual faculties.

Moreover, the education which is suited to the male, is

not calculated to render the female amiable and useful in society.

This is an observation of all times. The ancients were too good observers not to know that woman, by her lesser stature, her weaker organization, her predominant sensibility, and her peculiar function of multiplying the species, was not destined by nature to such toilsome labours as men.

We seek, accordingly, to develop in woman that modesty and gentleness which are proper to her, that soft and attractive air which characterizes her, and those seductive graces which distinguish her.

The constitution of women, indeed, bears only moderate exercise. Their feeble arms cannot support severe and long-continued labour. It renders them meagre, and deforms the organs, by compressing and destroying that cellular substance which contributes to the beauty of their outlines and of their complexion. The graces accommodate themselves little to labour, perspiration and sun-burning.

We must not, however, conclude from this, that females should be kept in a state of continual repose, or that the delicacy of their organization prevents their taking exercise.

It is a fact that labour, even the most excessive, is not so much to be feared as absolute idleness. The state of want which forces some women of the lowest class to perform labours that seem reserved for men, deprives them only of some attractions. Excessive indolence, on the contrary, destroys at once health, and that which women value more than health, though it never can subsist without it, namely beauty.

The more robust state of health in females brought up in the country is attributable to the exercise they enjoy.

Their movements are active and firm; their appetite is good, and their complexion florid; they are alert and gay; they know neither pain nor lassitude, although they are in action without cessation under all kinds of weather. It is exercise which gives them vigour, health and happiness – exercise to which they are so frequently subjected, even in infancy and youth.

We observe, also, that in a family where there are several sisters of similar constitution, the one who from circumstances has been accustomed to regular and daily exercise, almost always possesses most strength and vigour.

Mothers and teachers, therefore, instead of fearing that their children should fatigue themselves by exertion in active sports, should subject them early to it. They will thus give them more than merely life and instruction; they will confer on them health and strength.

But some mothers are afraid to see their daughters entering with spirit into exercises, and are of opinion that health cannot be obtained without sacrificing the graces which a female who is intended for society should possess.

They may rest assured that no recommender of exercise would endeavour to make a stout, robust woman of a little, delicate and nervous girl, or would prescribe for her the female gymnastics of the half-naked women of Lacedaemon, as instituted by Lycurgus.

What we can, and what we should endeavour to do, is to obtain a good constitution, absence from all deformity, and sufficient strength to prevent the display of vicious sensibility, but not to destroy that delicacy and those attractions which constitute beauty and grace.

But it may be feared that the peculiar structure and the natural weakness of woman, may render dangerous the exercises intended to combat it.

Those who make such objections should recollect that the circumstances which distinguish the sexes, and which modify them, remain imperfect and without action, until the age of puberty, and that children of both sexes have nearly the same appetites, the same wants, and the same inclinations. It is hence we recognize in them nearly the same physiognomy, a similar tone of voice, and similar manners.

This will be the less surprising when it is known that the internal organization, even the structure of the bones, has a greater resemblance in early life than at a subsequent period. Thus until they arrive at maturity, the pelvis, or basin, is rarely larger than in youths. Hence all the exercises which depend upon position and walking, will not be more difficult for them than for boys; while, for full-grown women, these exercises are more difficult and embarrassing.

This community of structure, as well as the fact that, at this early age, activity, restlessness and the desire of motion are remarkable in girls, all point out the danger of repose.

Instead, therefore, of being afraid of exercise for young girls, they should be subjected to it as soon as possible; and, when this is the case, they uniformly prove the truth of the observation, made by teachers of exercises, that females, in agility, precision and address, surpass boys of the same age.

So much for the effects of exercise upon the locomotive system.

With regard to the vital or nutritive system, it is not less certain that exercise augments the circulation and respiration, and perfects the formation of the blood and the nourishment of the body, in the same proportion in which the power of the lungs is developed.

By carrying towards the exterior the forces which, during a state of repose, tend almost always to concentrate themselves either in the brain or in the abdominal organs, exercise makes of these forces a more exact distribution, re-establishes or maintains their equilibrium, and, by exciting the circulation, provokes the insensible perspiration, without which health and beauty are impossible.

In relation to the diseases of this system, it is evident that, when the circulation is reanimated and accelerated, fewer engorgements of blood take place in the abdominal and inferior regions, and the inertia of chlorosis is dissipated.

In regard to the mental system, exercise, while it increases the activity of the muscles, prevents, as we have seen, the vicious predominance of the sensitive system. Diseased sensibility can never exist where the constitution has not been suffered to become enervated by indolence. When external agitation employs our faculties, the interior reposes.

If already the defective power of the mental functions tends to too vivid mobility, exercise gives them more of the stability of energy. The nervous susceptibility, which is increased by weakness, is reduced to its proper degree, as soon as exercise has strengthened the organs. By this useful diversion, the affections of the heart are calmed. '*Otia si tollas, periere Cupidinis arcus.*'

But this is not all: by diminishing the causes of exaggeration in the affections and passions, mildness and goodness, the most certain sources of happiness, remain in conjunction with health.

There can, therefore, be no doubt of the utility of exercise in remedying whatever may be defective in the female organization, and laying the foundation of a constitution exempt from infirmities and disease.

PART II

PARTICULAR EXERCISES

———————

OF THE KINDS OF EXERCISE

THE exercises called active are those in which the body is moved and agitated by its own force, with or without the particular influence and direction of the organs of sense.

These voluntary exercises always produce a general excitement more or less powerful.

The class called passive, or communicated exercises, are those in which the body is acted upon and moved by a cause distinct from muscular action, or without the muscles assisting in any other way than by a contraction merely sufficient to preserve a fixed position.

These exercises merely produce a succession of impulses in the living parts, calculated to brace and strengthen them without exciting.

Mixed exercises, such as riding on horseback, produce each of these results.

———————

PASSIVE EXERCISES

THESE, indeed, are not properly exercises, because the body is moved in them without effort; but as they are often employed as an introduction to active exercises, it would have been improper to omit a sort of preliminary notice of them.

Passive exercises have a remarkable effect upon nutrition: they increase the strength and vigour, without much excitement of the organs, raising no beatings of the heart, nor overheating, nor, generally speaking, producing perspiration.

Without enquiring by what means nutrition is, under their influence, performed with greater energy, and rendered more general, it may be observed that, thereby, the organs of which the body is composed, appear to experience, throughout their substance, a number of vibrations which may exercise the fibres, augment their density, and render them stronger.

While, in active exercises, nutrition is distributed so that the more certain parts are exercised, the more preponderance they acquire in relation to others which lose power in the same proportion; in passive exercises, on the contrary, distribution and nutrition exist in the most perfect equality.

FRICTION with the hand and with the flesh-brush, shampooing, &c. may be ranked with passive exercises.

In the SWING, if a second person gives the impulse, the exercise is purely passive; but if the person swinging assist in the action, or perform it alone, it has, in the same proportion, the effects of active exercise. This exercise, however, is dangerous, unless used with discretion: great care should be taken that the ropes are strong and well secured, and the seat fastened firmly.

SUSPENDED COUCHES form an exercise similar to swinging; the only difference being that the person exercised reclines, instead of sitting upright, and that the curve described in the motion is considerably less. This exercise is more especially useful in alleviating pain and in producing sleep.

SEE-SAW furnishes a succession of movements which are more powerful than the preceding. As it consists in balancing a plank, the centre of which rests upon a solid axis, one person being seated at each end, and one rising as the other descends, this exercise is not exactly passive; each party takes an active part, either to keep herself on, or to rise, by impelling the extremity of the lever when it strikes the ground.

SAILING, considered only as a movement communicated, has not so great an effect upon the functions as carriage exercise. The sailor experiences a succession of balancings, rather than shocks.

It nevertheless presents physical agents which produce a remarkable change in the constitution of sailors. These appear to be:

One. The sea-breeze, which, in the same degree of latitude, is much cooler than that of the land.

Two. The greater purity of the air at sea than on land. Although the ocean is inhabited by an immense number of living beings, the decomposition of their bodies does not appear to produce any putridity in the water, and they consequently produce none in the atmosphere which rests on its surface.

Three. The temperature of the surface of the sea, which is more uniform and less changeable than that on shore. The land, in some places, by means of its mountains and valleys, seems to concentrate and preserve immense quantities of solar heat, to which other places are, by their position, inaccessible. This cannot be the case at sea, where nothing interferes with the free course of caloric.

CARRIAGE EXERCISE produces greater motions, because the flooring upon which the feet rest necessarily receives the jolts and shocks which the wheels cause, owing to the roughness of the ground, and transmits them to the person within.

If the ground be very uneven, and the speed very great, the shocks may be so continual and violent, as to render this exercise insupportable and injurious to very weak constitutions. If the rate be slower and easily endured, it is evident that it may, in some cases, have beneficial effects upon the organs.

The refinement in building carriages, however, is carried so far that not only do the shocks received by the wheels no longer transmit any percussive motion to our organs, but even the most easy balancings scarcely reach us.

This mode of exercise in a carriage cannot consequently be of great utility in re-establishing a constitution enervated by luxury or study. It is calculated only to increase what is termed nervous susceptibility, to put us out of a condition to resist the most trifling collision, and to render us still more attentive to all the slight shades of disagreeable sensation.

The transmission of shocks being in indirect ratio to the elasticity of the springs, and direct to the tension of the braces, carriages of this kind, in which the springs are the least elastic, and the braces as tight as possible, appear to be the most suitable; for if, on one side, the line of motion should be sufficiently broken to avoid the rough shocks that a cart produces, on the other, it should not be sufficiently broken to annul the shocks which constitute precisely the advantage of this kind of exercise.

As carriage exercise gives more vigour to the organs, without adding to the activity of their functions, facilitates assimilation – without occasioning loss – and enjoys, in a very high degree, the advantages peculiar to passive exercises; it is, when necessary, suited to all ages, particularly to the two extremes of life, and is very favourable to the re-establishment of convalescents who cannot yet take any active exercise.

MIXED EXERCISES

MIXED exercises are composed of two orders of movement: the first is communicated to the individual by a foreign power; the second has its principle in the individual himself, and is not generally executed except to regulate the first.

The effects of these exercises are of course the same as the effects of passive exercises joined to active ones.

RIDING furnishes an example of what has just been stated.

In riding, the shock of the horse's feet upon the ground produces in the animal's body a percussive action, which shakes the rider. He undergoes a succession of lively shocks, of which the action is very extensive, if the horse be trotting, cantering, or galloping. If, on the contrary, the horse is walking slowly, the effects are very trifling.

Equitation is recommended to ladies in too general a manner, and is proper for them only under particular circumstances. When the health is not impaired, this exercise has many disadvantages, in the twist it gives the body; the raising of the shoulder; the enlargement of the size of the waist, by the exercise of its muscles in maintaining the balance; the deforming of the limbs; the rendering the voice coarse; the injury of the complexion; the unnatural consolidation of the bones of the lower part of the body; the improper irritation and subsequent debility it produces; the masculine air it bestows, &c. &c.

Roussel justly remarks, that ladies never derive, from riding, the same advantage as men; for, being compelled to indulge in it with precaution, they seem, in mounting on horseback, to lose those graces which are natural to them, without gaining those of the sex which they endeavour to imitate.

ACTIVE EXERCISES – OF POSITION

OF STANDING GENERALLY

BEFORE entering into a detail of exercises, it is necessary to attend to position.

A standing position is the action by which we keep ourselves up.

Indeed this state, in which the body appears to be in repose, is itself a sort of exercise; for it consists in a continued effort of many muscles. The explanation which we must give of it will somewhat facilitate that of walking.

Everyone has observed that during sleep, or in a fainting fit, the head inclines forward and falls upon the breast. This is in accordance with the laws of gravity; for the head, resting upon the first vertebra at a point of its base which is nearer its posterior than anterior part, cannot remain in an upright position, except by an effort of the muscles of the back of the neck: it is the cessation of this effort that causes it to fall forward.

The body also is unable to remain straight, without fatigue. The vertebral column being placed behind, all the organs contained by the chest and abdomen are suspended in front of it, and would force it to bend forward unless the strong muscles of the back held it back. A proof of this may be seen in pregnant women, who are compelled, in consequence of the anterior part of the body being heavier than usual, to keep the vertebral column more fixed, and even thrown backward.

The same observation may be made with regard to the pelvis, basin, or lowest part of the trunk, which, by its conformation, would bend forward upon the thighs, if not kept back by the great muscles that form the hips.

In front of the thighs again are the muscles which, by keeping the kneepan in position, are the means of preventing the knee from bending.

Lastly, the muscles forming the calves of the legs, by

contracting, are the means of preventing the ankles from bending.

Such is the general mechanism of the standing position. It is, therefore, as observed, a concurrence of efforts: almost all the extending muscles are in a state of contraction all the time that this position is maintained.

The consequence is a fatigue which cannot be endured for any great length of time. Hence, we see persons in a standing position rest the weight of their body, first on one foot, then on another, for the purpose of procuring momentary ease to certain muscles.

For this reason also, standing still is more fatiguing than walking, in which the muscles are alternately contracted, and extended.

A question of importance on this subject, is what position of the feet affords the greatest solidity in standing. Here it is sufficient to state the fact, that the larger the base of support, the firmer and more solid will the position be.

We now adopt, as a fundamental one, the military position, which has been found practically the best, by those who have nothing else to do but to walk.

FUNDAMENTAL POSITION

The equal squareness of the shoulders and body to the front is the first and great principle of position. The heels must be in a line, and closed; the knees straight; the toes turned out, with the feet forming an angle of sixty degrees; the arms hanging close to the body; the elbows turned in and close to the sides; the hands open to the front, with the view of preserving the elbow in the position above described;

the little fingers lightly touching the clothing of the limbs, with the thumb close to the forefingers; the belly rather drawn in, and the breast advanced, but without constraint; the body upright, but inclining forward, so that the weight of it may principally bear on the fore part of the feet; the head erect, and the eyes straight to the front.

To these brief directions, I must add that, in standing, the whole figure must be in such a position, that the ear, shoulder, haunch, knee and ankle are all in a line; that it must be stretched as much as possible, by raising the back of the head, drawing in the chin, straightening the spine, rising on the hips, and extending the legs; that the object of keeping the back thus straight is to allow of standing longer without fatigue; that it is important to expand the chest and to throw the shoulders back, with the shoulderblades or scapulae quite flat behind; and that though by men, in military instructions, the body is thus inclined forward in standing without arms, yet when these are assumed, the body is immediately thrown about two inches backward, into a nearly perpendicular position (Plate VIII. *fig.* 1).

This position, therefore, will be modified in standing at ease, in walking, and especially in ordinary walking; but it is an excellent fundamental position, and it cannot be too accurately acquired.

This is the amount of the drill sergeant's instructions as to position, though this last part is omitted in the Manual describing the field exercise and evolutions of the army.

Females find the standing position very fatiguing; however, it may be modified.

In consequence of the pelvis, basin, or lowest part of the

PLATE VIII

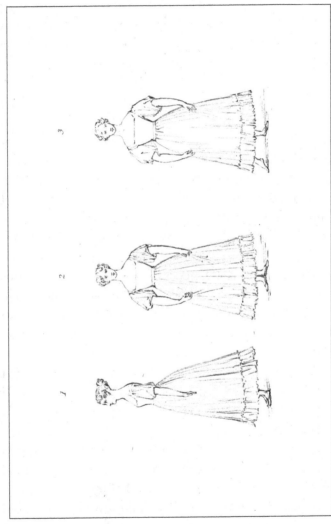

1   2   3

FUNDAMENTAL AND OTHER POSITIONS

body being larger in them than in man, the bones of the thighs are more separated above, and as they necessarily approach more closely below, this produces an inclination to be in-kneed. It is true the feet are not so close together as in men; but as they are smaller and do not so well support a standing position in front, where there is most need of support, it is, in fact, more difficult for women.

We may remark, however, that the pelvis not being developed before the age of puberty, the standing position of young girls is the same as in youths.

What has now been said regards the general position of the whole figure; and to this the more particular positions of the feet, which are the elements of dancing, are properly a sequel. Both, therefore, on their own account and for the sake of what follows, must be next described. It is of great importance that they be thoroughly understood and accurately and easily performed.

POSITIONS IN DANCING

In all these positions, the body should be kept perfectly erect; the shoulders thrown back, and the bust advanced; the arms rounded; the forefinger and thumb occupied in holding out the dress; the other fingers neatly grouped.

The first position is formed by placing the heels together and throwing the toes back, so that the feet form a straight line.

In the first attempts at this position, the toes should not be more turned out than will admit of the body maintaining its proper balance: they must be brought to the correct position only by degrees, until the pupil can place the feet,

PLATE IX

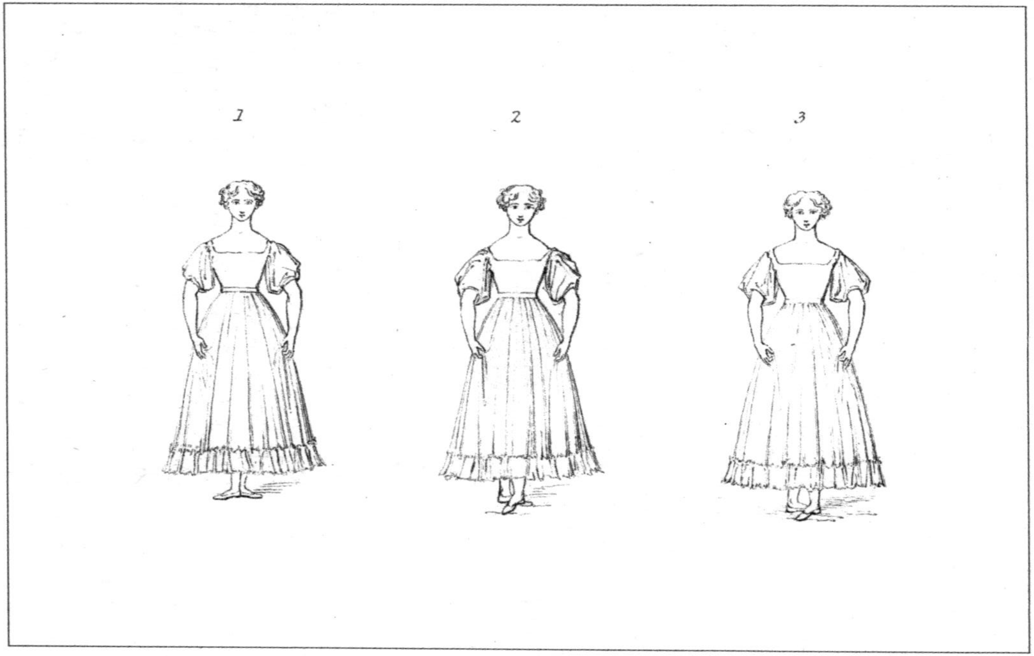

POSITIONS IN DANCING

heel to heel, in a straight line, without affecting the steadiness of the body or arms (Plate VIII. *fig.* 2).

The second position is formed by moving the right foot sideways, from the first position to about the distance of its own length from the heel of the left.

Of the foot thus placed, the heel must be raised, so that the toes alone rest on the ground; the instep being bent as much as possible, and the foot retaining its primitive direction outward.

In this case, as in the first, the foot should be brought by degrees correctly to perform this action; and the toes should be gradually thrown back as far as the pupil's power to preserve her balance will permit (Plate VIII. *fig.* 3).

The third position is formed by drawing the right foot from the second position, to about the middle of the front of the left; the feet being kept close to each other, so that the heel of one foot is brought to the ankle of the other, and seems to lock in with it: thus the feet are nearly half crossed.

In drawing the right foot into this position, its heel must be brought to the ground as it approaches the left, and kept forward during its progress, so that the toe may retain its proper direction outward (Plate IX. *fig.* 1).

The fourth position is formed by moving the foot about its own length forward from the third position, keeping the heel forward, and the toe backward, during the progress of the foot; and it must be so placed as to be exactly opposite to the other heel, or rather to the centre of the left foot, so that the feet half cross without touching.

In moving the right foot forward, the toe may be slightly raised (Plate IX. *fig.* 2).

The fifth position is formed by drawing the right foot back from the fourth position, so that its heel is brought close to the toes of the left foot, the feet being completely crossed.

The right heel, in this position, is gradually brought to the ground as it approaches the left foot, precisely as in formerly drawing the left foot from the second to the third (Plate IX. *fig.* 3).

In all these positions, the left foot is to retain its primitive situation.

In all these positions, also, the knees may be bent without raising the heels in the least from the ground; and to give flexibility and strength to the instep, they should be often practised on the toes.

———

EXTENSION MOTIONS

IN order to supple the figure, open the chest, and give freedom to the muscles of soldiers, the first three movements of the extension motions, as laid down for the sword exercise, are ordered to be practised.

It is, indeed, truly observed that too many methods cannot be used to improve the carriage, and banish a rustic air; but the greatest care must be taken not to throw the body backward instead of forward, as being contrary to every true principle of movement.

I accordingly here introduce these extension motions, as not less valuable to ladies than to men, adding the fourth and fifth, and prefixing to each the respective word of command, in order that they may be the more distinctly and accurately executed.

Attention. The body is to be erect, the heels close together, and the hands hanging down on each side.

First Extension Motion. This serves as a caution, and the motion tends to expand the chest, raise the head, throw back the shoulders, and strengthen the muscles of the back.

One. Bring the hands and arms to the front, the fingers lightly touching at the points, and the nails downwards; then raise them in a circular direction well above the head, the ends of the fingers still touching, the thumbs pointing to the rear, the elbows pressed back, and the shoulders kept down (Plate X. *fig.* 1).

Two. Separate and extend the arms and fingers, forcing them obliquely back, till they come extended on a line with the shoulders; and, as they fall gradually thence to the original position of Attention, endeavour, as much as possible, to elevate the neck and chest.

These two motions should be frequently practised, with the head turned as much as possible to the right or left, and the body kept square to the front: this tends very materially to supple the neck, &c.

Three. Turn the palms of the hands to the front, pressing back the thumbs with the arms extended, and raise them to the rear, till they meet above the head; the fingers pointing upwards, with the ends of the thumbs touching (Plate X. *fig.* 2).

Four. Keep the arms and knees straight, and bend over from the hips till the hands touch the feet, the head being brought down in the same direction (Plate X. *fig.* 3).

Five. With the arms flexible and easy from the shoulders,

PLATE X

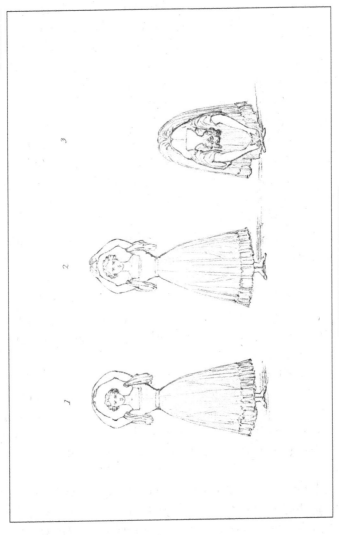

EXTENSION MOTIONS

PLATE XI

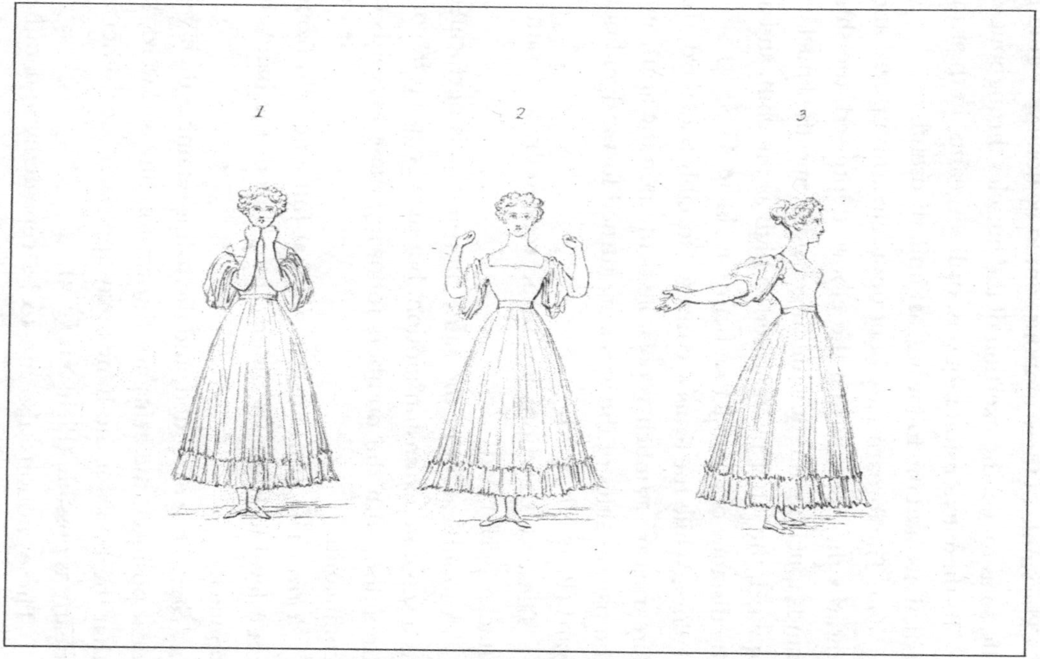

EXTENSION MOTIONS

raise the body gradually, so as to resume the position of Attention.

The whole of these motions should be done very gradually, so as to feel the exertion of the muscles throughout.

To these extension motions, drill sergeants, in their instructions, add the following, as similarly useful.

One. The forearms are bent upon the arms upward and towards the body, having the elbows depressed, the shut hands touching on the little finger sides, and the knuckles upward, the latter being raised as high as the chin, and at the distance of about a foot before it (Plate XI. *fig.* 1).

Two. While the arms are thrown forcibly backward, the forearms are as much as possible bent upon the arms, and the palmar sides of the wrists are turned forward and outward (Plate XI. *fig.* 2).

These two motions are to be repeatedly and rather quickly performed.

A modification of the same movements is performed as a separate extension motion, but may be given in continuation, with the numbers following these as words of command.

Three. The arms are extended at full length in front, on a level with the shoulders, the palms of the hands in contact.

Four. Thus extended, and the palms retaining their vertical position, the arms are thrown forcibly backward, so that the backs of the hands may approach each other as nearly as possible (Plate XI. *fig.* 3).

These motions also are to be repeatedly and rather quickly performed.

Another extension motion, similarly added, consists in swinging the right arm in a circle, in which, beginning from the pendent position, the arm is carried upward in front, by the side of the head, and downward behind, the object being, in the latter part of this course, to throw it as directly backward as possible. The same is then done with the left arm. Lastly, both arms are thus exercised together.

These motions are performed quickly.

THE EXERCISE WITH THE ROD

THE rod for this purpose should be light, smooth, inflexible, and need not be more than three or four feet in length.

FIRST EXERCISE

The rod is first grasped near the extremities by the two hands, the thumbs being inward.

Without changing the position of the hands on the rod, it is then brought to a vertical position: the right hand being uppermost holds it above the head, the left is against the lower part of the body.

By an opposite movement, the right hand is lowered and the left raised.

This change is executed repeatedly and quickly.

SECOND EXERCISE

From the first position of the rod, it is raised over the head;

PLATE XII

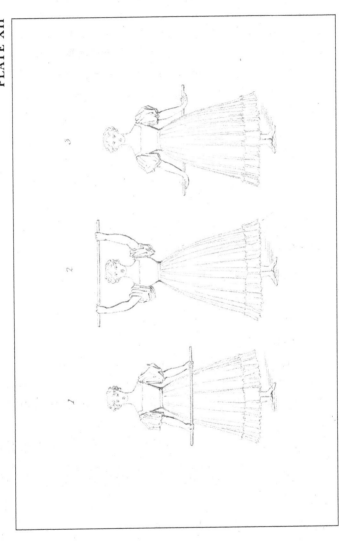

EXERCISES WITH THE ROD

and, in doing so, the closer the hands are, the better will be the effect upon the shoulder.

It is afterwards carried behind the back, holding so firmly that no change takes place in the position of the hands.

This movement is then reversed, to bring it back over the head to the first position.

THIRD EXERCISE

The same exercises are performed by grasping the rod with the hands in an opposite position; that is to say, with the thumbs in front or the palms of the hands forward (Plate XII. *fig.* 1).

It is raised parallel with the shoulders, extending it first on the left and then on the right arm.

FOURTH EXERCISE

The rod is next raised above the head, the hands being still in their new position (Plate XII. *fig.* 2).

It is afterwards lowered behind the back (Plate XII. *fig.* 3).

The exercise is concluded by bringing the rod to its original position in front.

———————

These exercises cannot be performed in all their different movements with promptitude and regularity without many trials and repetitions. Their tendency is to confirm

the good position and the flexibility of the shoulders, produced by the extension motions.

THE DUMB-BELLS

THIS instrument is one of the oldest used in gymnastics. It
may be seen in the Latin work of *Mercurialis de Arte Gym-
nastica*; and though its form was not precisely the same as
at present, the result produced was similar. It has been long
in use in England, where it enters into the school exercise
of most seminaries for the instruction of ladies.

For children from six to ten years of age, dumb-bells
should not weigh more than from three to four pounds
each; and for children from ten to fifteen years of age, they
may weigh from four to six pounds each.

To use dumb-bells with all the advantage they admit of,
the young person should stand in the fundamental position
already described.

To obtain the first position, the hands and the dumb-
bells are, by a slight rotatory movement of the arm outward
and backward, brought behind the lower part of the body,
so as to make the two extremities of the dumb-bells next to
the little fingers touch each other.

The fingers in this case touch the muscles of the hips,
and the back of the hand is outward (Plate XIII. *fig.* 1).

FIRST EXERCISE

In the first exercise from this position, a regular motion

PLATE XIII

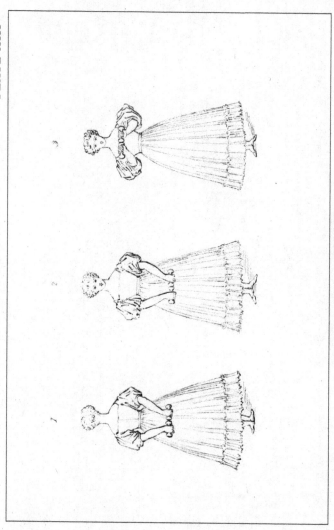

EXERCISES WITH DUMB-BELLS

PLATE XIV

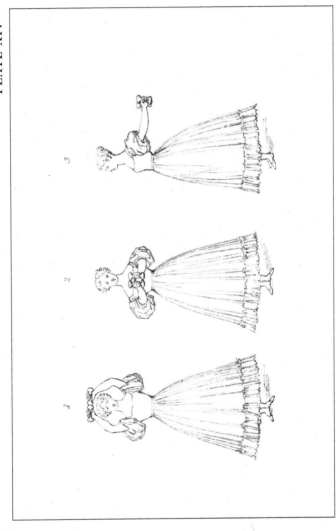

EXERCISES WITH DUMB-BELLS

is commenced, which consists in giving to the depending and extended arms, at the same time, a circular and rotatory movement, forward and inward, to the front of the body, so that the dumb-bells perform each a semicircle (Plate XIII. *fig.* 2), making a complete circle between them, but with this difference in position, that when they are behind, they touch at the exterior extremities, or those on the side of the little finger, and when they are in front of the thighs, they touch at the other extremities.

SECOND EXERCISE

In the second exercise, from the same position, the hands are raised together towards the front and middle of the chest, and approximated, so that the ball on the thumb-side of one dumb-bell may touch that of the other (Plate XIII. *fig.* 3). With the arms extended, they are then allowed to drop with sufficient force to swing them round the body to the first position. This is repeated several times.

THIRD EXERCISE

In the third exercise, from the same position, the arms are raised above the head, and the dumb-bells are made to touch at their extremities, being kept in a horizontal position (Plate XIV. *fig.* 1). The hands are then allowed to fall gently into the first position.

FOURTH EXERCISE

In the fourth exercise, the arms are stretched out straight

from the shoulders (Plate XIV. *fig.* 2) and the hands are moved horizontally backward (Plate XIV. *fig.* 3) and forward, the dumb-bells being in a vertical position.

———————

This employment of the dumb-bells should not at first be persisted in longer than a minute or two at a time, but the duration of each succeeding exercise may be gradually increased.

N.B. Until the introduction of the Indian sceptres, or Indian clubs, this exercise was valuable, notwithstanding the inconvenient jerks which it communicates to the shoulders. It should now be superseded by that exercise, which is incomparably more varied, graceful, and beneficial.

———————

THE INDIAN SCEPTRE EXERCISE

THE PORTION PRACTISED WITH CLUBS IN THE ARMY

One. A sceptre is held by the handle, pendent on each side (Plate XV. *fig.* 1); that in the right hand is carried over the head and left shoulder until it hangs perpendicularly on the right side of the spine (Plate XV. *fig.* 2); that in the left hand is carried over the former, in exactly the opposite direction (see the same figure), until it hangs on the opposite side; holding both sceptres still pendent, the hands are raised somewhat higher than the head (Plate XV. *fig.* 3);

PLATE XV

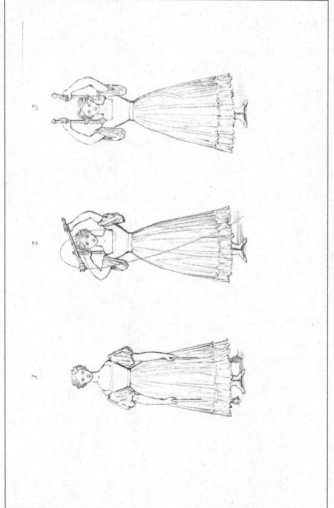

INDIAN SCEPTRE EXERCISE

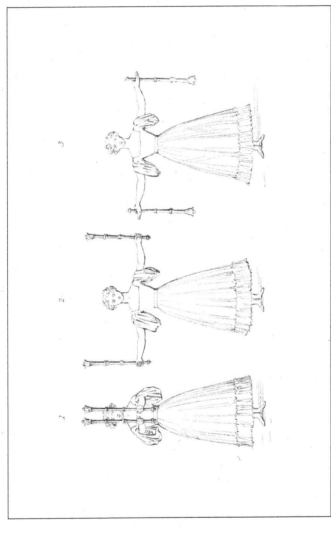

PLATE XVI

INDIAN SCEPTRE EXERCISE

PLATE XVII

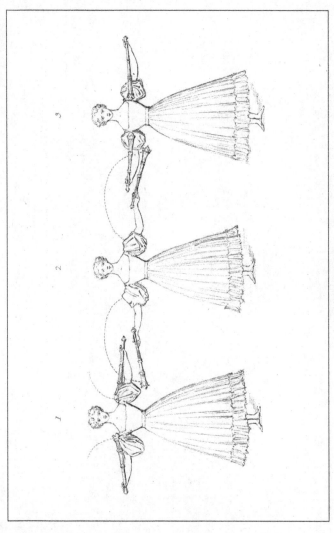

INDIAN SCEPTRE EXERCISE

PLATE XVIII

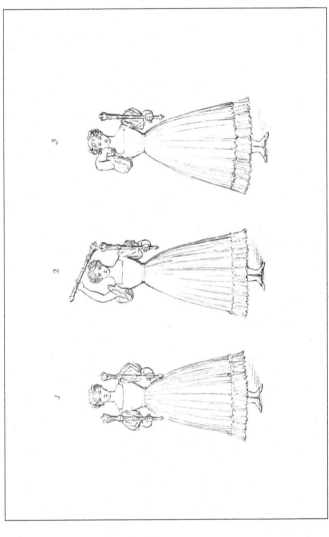

INDIAN SCEPTRE EXERCISE

PLATE XIX

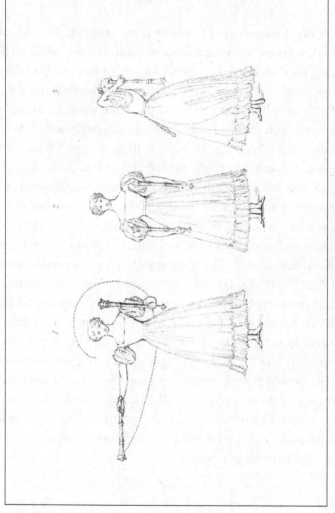

INDIAN SCEPTRE EXERCISE

with the sceptres in the same position, both arms are extended outward and backward (Plate XVI. *fig.* 3); they are, lastly, dropped into the first position. All this is done slowly.

Two. Commencing from the same position, the ends of both sceptres are swung upward until they are held, vertically and side by side, at arm's length, in front of the body, the hands being as high as the shoulders (Plate XVI. *fig.* 1); they are next carried in the same position, at arm's length, and on the same level, as far backward as possible (Plate XVI. *fig.* 2); each is then dropped backward until it hangs vertically downward (Plate XVI. *fig.* 3); and this exercise ends as the first. Previous, however, to dropping the sceptres backward, it greatly improves this exercise, by a turn of the wrist upward and backward, to carry the sceptres into a horizontal position behind the shoulders, so that if long enough, their ends would touch (Plate XVII. *fig.* 1); next, by a turn of the wrist outward and downward, to carry them horizontally outward (Plate XVII. *fig.* 2); then by a turn of the wrist upward and forward, to carry them into a horizontal position before the breast (Plate XVII. *fig.* 3); again, to carry them horizontally outward; and, finally, to drop them backward; and thence to the first position. All this is also done slowly.

Three. The sceptres are to be swung by the sides, first separately, and then together, exactly as the hands were in the last extension motion.

PLATE XX

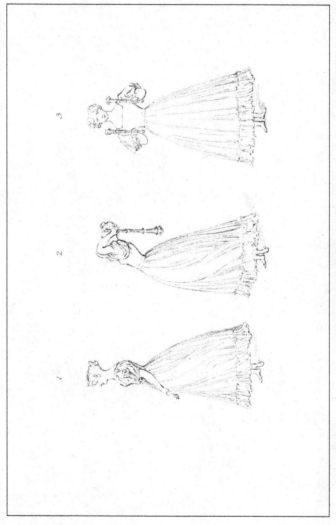

INDIAN SCEPTRE EXERCISE

PLATE XXI

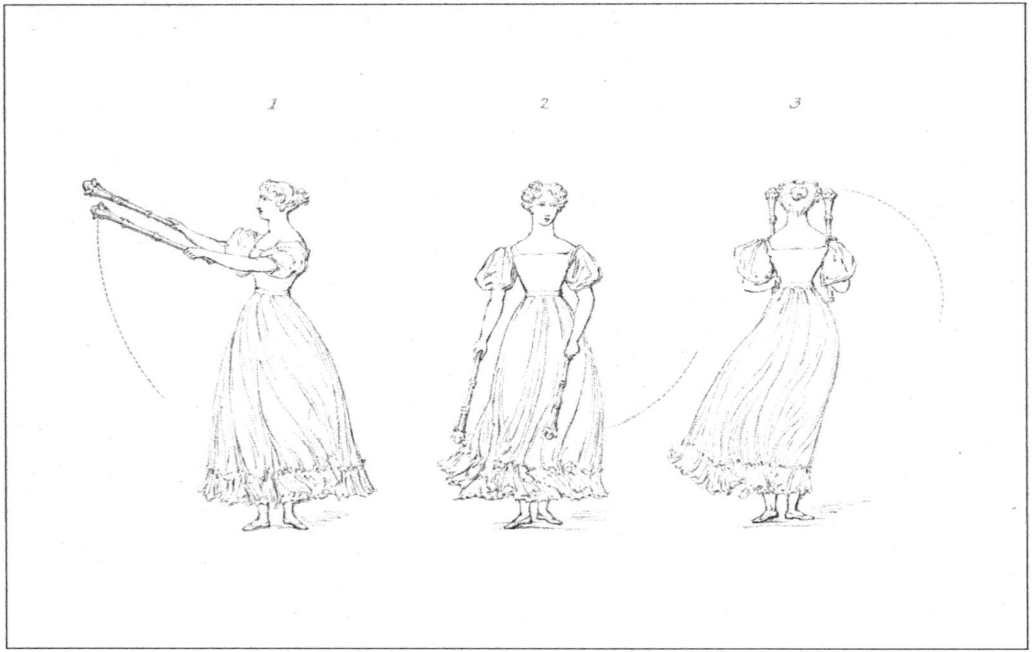

INDIAN SCEPTRE EXERCISE

THE NEW AND MORE BEAUTIFUL PORTION NOW ADDED FROM THE INDIAN PRACTICE

One. The sceptres are held upright in front of the body, the elbows being near the haunches, and the forearms horizontal (Plate XVIII. *fig.* 1); the sceptre in the right hand is then carried over the head and left shoulder (Plate XVIII. *fig.* 2), dropping as low as possible behind (Plate XVIII. *fig.* 3), and returning to its first position; the same is done with the left hand; then with the right; and so on with each alternately. All this is performed with a swinging motion, so that the end of each sceptre describes a circle which commences before the head, descends obliquely backward, and ascends again.

Two. After carrying the sceptre in the right hand from the same position around the head and left shoulder, as already described, it is stretched horizontally outward by the extended arm (Plate XIX. *fig.* 1); and thence returned to the first position; the same is then done with the left hand; and so on with each alternately. The swing is here broken by the lateral extension.

Three. The sceptres, held chiefly between the thumb and first and second fingers, rest on the fronts of the arms extended downward and slightly forward, and reach somewhat obliquely from the thumb and now inner side of the hands, of which the backs are turned forward, to the outsides of the shoulders (Plate XIX. *fig.* 2); that held in the right hand is then thrown over the shoulder and hangs downward behind it, while the whole of that side of the body is turned forward, the back and neck bent, so that the chin is raised and the chest thrown upward (Plate XIX. *fig.* 3), and, as the body is again turned to the front, that sceptre is drawn over the shoulder and brought to its first position; at the moment in which the body reaches the front, however, the same begins to be done with the left hand; and so on with each alternately.

Four. This differs from the second only in this respect, that the arms no longer act distinctly, but together; their motions being blended by the left commencing as soon as the right has made its circle round the head, and forming its own circle while the right is extending, and so on with regard to each. This explanation, and a reference to the description and plates illustrating the first and second exercise, make this quite plain.

Five. This differs from the third chiefly in this, that the arms no longer act distinctly, but together; both sceptres, however, being kept down until the lateral turn is complete (Plate XX. *fig.* 1), both being then thrown over the shoulders at once, with the back and neck bent (Plate XX. *fig.* 2), and both returning gradually (Plate XX. *fig.* 3) over the shoulders as the body passes to the opposite side.

Six. This is an exercise in which the lady crosses the apartment from side to side. The first exercise is here performed once with each arm, commencing with the arm of the side towards which the freer space permits her most readily to go. (See description and plates illustrating the first exercise.) Supposing this to be to the right of her first position, on finishing the second circle of the first exercise, namely that with the left arm, and bringing it in front, both sceptres, being thrown to the right side (Plate XXI. *fig.* 1), are swung with extended arms to the left, sweeping in a circle downward in front of the feet (Plate XXI. *fig.* 2). The left foot being at that moment lifted to perform a wheel backward upon the right toe, the face is turned opposite to its first direction, ground being gained by the left foot placing itself towards what was originally the right side, and the ends of the sceptres, without the slightest pause, continue their sweep upward to their first position (Plate XXI. *fig.* 3). The same is only repeated; the lady remembering always to commence with the arm of the side to which she means to advance.

THE POSITION IN WALKING

IN all walking, the position is nearly the same, namely, that already described but modified by progression.

PROPER POSITION

The head should be upright, easy, and capable of free motion, right, left, up, or down, without affecting the position of the body. The body must be kept erect and square to the front, having the breast projected, and the stomach retracted, though not so as to injure either freedom of respiration, or ease of attitude. The shoulders should be kept moderately and equally back and low; and the arms should hang unconstrainedly by the sides. The balance on the limbs must be perfect. The knees should be straight, and the toes turned out as described. The weight of the body should be somewhat thrown forward, as this facilitates progression.

But though, in progression, the weight of the body should be thrown somewhat forward, it must be understood that this requires a voluntary effort, and consequently a kind of occupation of the mind, with the mere mechanical act of progression. This inclination of the body is, therefore, unfavourable to thought, conversation, and the expression of emotion and passion by natural gesture.

The moment, therefore, that these occupations of the mind occur, as in all walking for reflexion or conversation, the body falls naturally into the upright position, and is placed more or less at ease from the inclination and restraint which are necessary in progression.

Hence it is that vain and imbecile creatures, incapable of thought, as the lads who become officers merely to wear a red coat with tinsel upon it, may in a moment be known by their senses and their will being evidently always and altogether directed to their manner of walking and to the adjustment of their persons. Such people are always weak-minded and worthless in all the duties of human life.

MILITARY POSITION

The military position in walking does not essentially differ from this, except in points that exclusively regard the soldier: as that the head be kept well up and straight to the front, and the eyes not turned to the right or left; the arms and hands kept perfectly steady by the sides, and on no account suffered to move or vibrate; care, however, being taken that the hand does not cling to the thighs, or partake in the least degree of the movement of the limbs.

THE BALANCE STEP

THE object of this is to teach the free movement of the limbs, preserving at the same time perfect squareness of shoulders, with the utmost steadiness of body, and no labour is spared to attain this first and most essential object, which forms indeed the very foundation of good walking.

The instructor must be careful that a habit is not contracted of drooping or throwing back a shoulder at these motions, which are intended practically to show the true principles of walking, and that steadiness of body is compatible with perfect freedom in the limbs.

WITHOUT GAINING GROUND

To ensure precision, the military words of command are prefixed.

Caution. Balance step without gaining ground, commencing with the left foot.

Front. The left foot is brought gently forward with the toe at the proper angle, the foot about three inches from the ground, the left heel in line with the toe of the right foot.

Rear. When steady, the left foot is brought gently back (without a jerk), the left knee a little bent, the left toe brought close to the right heel. The left foot in this position will not be so flat as when in front, as the toe will be a little depressed.

When steady, the words Front and Rear will be given alternately, and repeated to the rear three or four times.

To prevent fatigue, the word Halt will be given, when the left foot, either advanced, or to the rear, will be brought to the right.

The instructor will afterwards cause the balance to be made upon the left foot, advancing and retiring the right in the same manner.

GAINING GROUND

Front. On the word Front, the left foot is brought smartly to the front as before; the knee being straight, and the toe turned out a little to the left and remaining about three inches from the ground. This posture is continued for a few seconds only in the first instance, till practice gives steadiness in the position.

Forward. On this word, the left foot is brought to the ground, at 30 inches from heel to heel, while the right foot is raised at the same moment, and continues extended to the rear. The body remains upright, but inclining forward; the head erect, and neither turned to the right nor left.

Two. On the word Two, the right foot is brought forward in a line with the left, the toe a little turned out, and the sole quite flat, but raised two inches from the ground.

Front. On the word Front, the right foot is brought forward, and so on.

WALKING

WALKING IN GENERAL

OF all exercises, walking is the most simple and easy. The weight of the body rests on one foot while the other is advanced; it is then thrown upon the advanced foot while the other is brought forward; and so on in succession.

In this mode of progression, the slowness and equal distribution of motion is such that many muscles are employed in a greater or lesser degree; each acts in unison with the rest; and the whole remains compact and united. Hence, the time of its movements may be quicker or slower, without deranging the union of the parts, or the equilibrium of the whole.

It is owing to these circumstances, that walking displays so much of the character of the walker, that it is light and gay in women and children, steady and grave in men and elderly persons, irregular in the nervous and irritable, measured in the affected and formal, brisk in the sanguine, heavy in the phlegmatic, and proud or humble, bold or timid, &c., in strict correspondence with individual character.

The utility of walking exceeds that of all other modes of progression. While the able pedestrian is independent of stage-coaches and hired horses, he alone fully enjoys the scenes through which he passes, and is free to dispose of his time as he pleases.

To counterbalance these advantages, greater fatigue is doubtless attendant on walking: but this fatigue is really the result of previous inactivity; for daily exercise, gradually increased, by rendering walking more easy and agreeable,

PLATE XXII

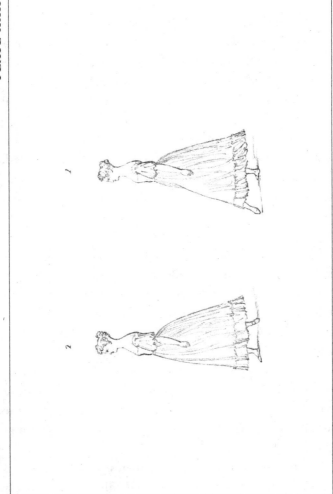

WALKING – THE SLOW WALK

and inducing its more frequent practice, diminishes fatigue in such a degree, that very great distances may be accomplished with pleasure, instead of painful exertion.

In relation to health, walking accelerates respiration and circulation, increases the temperature and cutaneous exhalation, and excites appetite and healthful nutrition. Hence, as an anonymous writer observes, the true pedestrian, after a walk of twenty miles, comes in to breakfast with freshness on his countenance, healthy blood coursing in every vein, and vigour in every limb, while the indolent and inactive man, having painfully crept over a mile or two, returns to a dinner which he cannot digest.

A firm, yet easy and graceful walk, however, is by no means common. There are few men who walk well, if they have not learnt to regulate their motions by the lessons of a master; and this instruction is still more necessary for ladies.

Having now, therefore, taken a general view of the character and utility of walking, I subjoin some more particular remarks on the following.

GENERAL MECHANISM OF WALKING

For the purpose of walking, we first bear upon one leg the weight of the body, which pressed equally on both. The other leg is then raised, and the foot quits the ground by rising from the heel to the point. For that purpose, the leg must be bent upon the thigh, and the thigh upon the pelvis: the foot is then carried straight forward, at a sufficient height to clear the ground without grazing it. To render it possible, however, to move this foot, the haunch which rested with its weight upon the thigh must turn forward and outward. As soon as, by this movement, this foot has passed the other, it must be extended on the leg, and the leg upon the thigh. In this manner, by the lengthening of the whole member, and without being drawn back, it reaches the ground at a distance in advance of the other foot, which is more considerable according to the length of the step. It is then placed so softly on the ground as not to jerk or shake the body in the slightest degree. As soon as the foot which has been placed on the ground becomes firm, the weight of the body is transported to the limb on that side, and the other foot, by a similar mechanism, is brought forward in its turn.

In all walking, the most important circumstances are, firstly, that the body must incline somewhat forward; and, secondly, that the movement of the leg and thigh must spring from the haunch, and be directed straight forward in a free and natural manner.

Walking may be performed in three different times – slow, moderate, or quick, which somewhat modify its action.

THE SLOW WALK, OR MARCH

In the march, the weight of the body is advanced from the heel to the instep, and the toes are most turned out. This being done, one foot, the left for instance, is advanced, with the knee straight, and the toe inclined to the ground, which, without being drawn back, it touches before the heel; in such a manner, however, that the sole, towards the conclusion of the step, is nearly parallel with the ground, which it next touches with its outer edge; the right foot is then immediately raised from the inner edge of the

PLATE XXIII

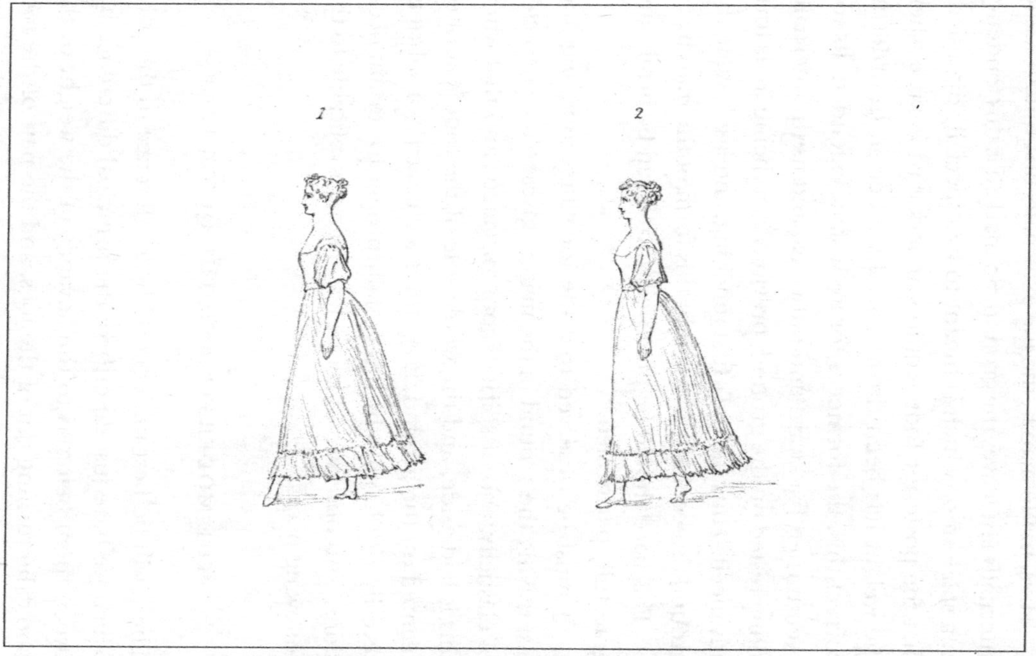

WALKING – THE MODERATE PACE

toe, and similarly advanced, inclined, and brought to the ground; and so in succession (Plate XXII. *figs.* 1 and 2).

Thus, in the march, the toe externally first touches, and internally last leaves the ground. So marked is this tendency in a stage step (which is meant to be especially dignified) that the posterior foot acquires an awkward flexure when the weight has been thrown on the anterior. In order to correct this, the former is for an instant extended, its toe even turned backward and outwards, and its tip internally alone rested on the ground, previous to its being in its turn advanced. Thus the toe's first touching, and last leaving the ground, is peculiarly marked in this form of the march.

This pace should be practised until it can be firmly and gracefully performed.

It must be observed that the toe's first touching and last leaving the ground in the march, gives to it a character of elasticity, and of spirit, vigour, or gaiety; and that when this is laid aside, and the whole sole of the foot is at once planted on the ground, it acquires a character of sobriety, severity, or gloom, which is equally proper to certain occasions. This observation is in a less degree applicable to the following paces.

THE MODERATE AND THE QUICK PACE

These will be best understood by a reference to the pace which we have just described; the principal difference between them being as to the advance of the weight of the body, the turning out of the toes, and the part of the foot which first touches and last leaves the ground.

We shall find that the times of these two paces require

PLATE XXIV

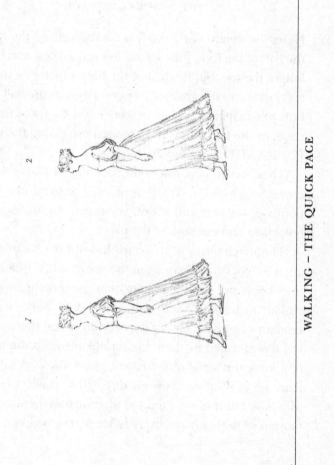

WALKING – THE QUICK PACE

a further advance of the weight, and suffer successively less and less of turning out the toes, and of this extended touching with the toe, and covering the ground with the foot.

THE MODERATE PACE

Here, the weight of the body is advanced from the heel to the ball of the foot; the toes are less turned out; and it is no longer the toe, but the ball of the foot, which first touches and last leaves the ground; its outer edge, or the ball of the little toe, first breaking the descent of the foot; and its inner edge, or the ball of the great toe last projecting the weight (Plate XXIII. *figs.* 1 and 2).

Thus, in this step, less of the foot may be said actively to cover the ground; and this adoption of nearer and stronger points of support and action is essential to the increased quickness and exertion of the pace.

The mechanism of this pace has not been sufficiently attended to. People pass from the march to the quick pace, they know not how; and hence all the awkwardness and embarrassment of their walk when their pace becomes moderate, and the misery they endure when this pace has to be performed by them unaccompanied, up the middle of a long and well-lighted room, where the eyes of a brilliant assembly are exclusively directed to them. Let those who have felt this but attend to what we have here said: the motion of the arms and every other part depend on it.

THE QUICK PACE

Here, the weight of the body is advanced from the heel

to the toes; the toes are least turned out; and still nearer and stronger points of support and action are chosen. The outer edge of the heel first touches the ground, and the sole of the foot projects the weight.

These are essential to the increased quickness of this pace (Plate XXIV. *figs.* 1 and 2).

It is important to remark, as to all these paces, that the weight is successively more thrown forward, and the toes are successively less turned out. In the theatrical form of the march, previously alluded to, the toes, as we have seen, are, in the posterior foot, though but for a moment, even thrown backward; in the moderate pace, they have an inter-mediate direction; and in the quick pace, they are thrown directly forward (Plates XXII, XXIII, and XXIV).

It is this direction of the toes, and still more the nearer and stronger points of support and action, namely, the heel and sole of the foot, which are essential to the quick pace so universally practised, but which, together with the greater inclination of the body, being ridiculously transferred to the moderate pace, make unfortunate people look so awk-ward as we shall now explain.

The time of the moderate pace is, as it were, filled up by the more complicated process of the step – by the gradual and easy breaking of the descent of the foot on its outer edge or the ball of the little toe, by the deliberate positing of the foot, by its equally gradual and easy projection from its inner edge or the ball of the great toe. The quick pace, if its time be lengthened, has no such filling up: the man stumps at once down on his heel, and could rise instantly from his sole, but finds that, to fill up his time, he must pause an instant; he feels that he should do something, and does not know what; his hands suffer the same momentary paralysis as his feet; he gradually becomes confused and embarrassed; deeply sensible of this, he at last exhibits it externally; a smile or a titter arises, though people do not well know at what; but, in short, the man has walked like a clown, because the mechanism of his step has not filled up its time, or answered its purpose.

———————

In the general walking of ladies, the step ought not to exceed the length of the foot; the leg should be put forward, without stiffness, in about the fourth position; but without any effort to turn the foot out, as it throws the body awry, and gives the person the appearance of a professional dancer; the arms should fall in their natural position, and all their movements and oppositions to the feet should be easy and unconstrained; and the pace should be neither too slow nor too quick.

The gait should be in harmony with the person – natural and tranquil, without giving the appearance of difficulty in advancing; and active, without the appearance of being in a hurry.

Nothing can be more ridiculous than a little woman, who takes innumerable minute steps with great rapidity, to get on with greater speed, except it be a tall woman, who throws out long legs as though she would dispute the road with the horses.

———————

I trust that the mechanism and time of the three paces, are here, for the first time, simply, clearly, and impressively described. I have not seen them rightly described elsewhere, which I think discreditable to the people whose business it is to teach such things. It becomes, indeed, of real importance among certain classes of society, and in certain situations; and I should be unworthy of my name, if I neglected it.

The following is the more imperfect, but, for practice, still useful, military description, with its words of command.

SLOW STEP

March. On the word March, the left foot is carried thirty inches to the front, and, without being drawn back, is placed softly on the ground, so as not to jerk or shake the body; seventy-five of these steps to be taken in a minute.

(The recruit is ordered to be carefully trained, and thoroughly instructed in this step, as an essential foundation for arriving at accuracy in the paces of more celerity. This is the slowest step at which troops are to move.)

QUICK STEP

The cadence of the slow pace having become perfectly habitual, a quick time is next taught, which is 108 steps in a minute, each of 30 inches, making 270 feet in a minute.

Quick March. The command Quick March being given with a pause between them, the word Quick is to be considered as a caution, and the whole must remain perfectly steady. On the word March, the whole move off, conforming to the direction already given.

(This pace is applied generally to all movements by large as well as small bodies of troops; and therefore the recruit is trained and thoroughly instructed in this essential part of his duty.)

DOUBLE MARCH

The directions for the march apply, in a great degree, to this step, which is 150 steps in the minute, each of 36 inches, making 450 feet in a minute.

Double March. On the word Double March, the whole step off together with the left feet; keeping the head erect, and the shoulders square to the front; the knees are a little bent; the body is more advanced than in the other marches; the arms hang with ease down the outside of the thigh. The person marching is carefully habituated to the full pace of 36 inches, otherwise he gets into the habit of a short trot, which defeats the obvious advantages of this degree of march.

In the army, great advantage attends the constant use of the plummet; and the several lengths swinging the times of the different marches in a minute, are as follows:

		In Hun
Slow time, 75 steps in the minute	· · · ·	· 24,96
Quick time, 108	· · · · · ·	· 12,03
Double march, 150	· · · · · ·	· 6,26

A musket-ball suspended by a string which is not subject to stretch, and on which are marked the different required lengths, answers the above purpose, may be easily acquired, and is directed to be frequently compared with an accurate standard in the adjutant's possession. The length of the plummet is to be measured from the point of suspension to the centre of the ball.

In practising all these paces, the pupils should also be accustomed to march upon a narrow plane, where there is room for only one foot, upon rough uneven ground, and on soft ground which yields to the foot, &c.

PARTICULAR UTILITY OF WALKING

Walking attracts the fluids to the inferior members more than to the upper, to which it gives little strength.

It is wrong, however, to assert that this exercise moves only the inferior parts of the body, while all the superior parts remain at rest; and that the liquids, to which the first have given a brisk impulse, must experience from the others a considerable resistance, which renders their course little uniform, and their distribution unequal.

Walking is not an exercise of the lower members only. The pelvis, as we have shown, moves from side to side as well as the body, so as to throw the weight upon the limb which is firm on the ground. This movement is more decided, according to the size of the pelvis. For this reason, children, in whom the pelvis is narrower, walk better than men; whilst, in females, the distance between the thigh bones renders walking more difficult, though they take very small steps. The arms also move alternately with the legs. But all these movements follow each other, and can, as we know, be repeated for a long time without fatigue, because the muscles which are exercised are sometimes in repose and sometimes in contraction.

Notwithstanding this, walking is less a sufficient employment of the muscles, than a kind of repose and relaxation. Moderate walking, indeed, exercises the very gentlest influence over all the functions.

Walking on a smooth, soft surface is an exercise that may be followed without inconvenience, and even with advantage after meals. The circumstance under which it may be most beneficial, is in convalescence, or when suffering under the fatigue of a forced exercise of the intellectual faculties.

If, however, we walk purely by regimen, the walk, not interesting us sufficiently to carry us out of ourselves, permits us to think too much of the motive which causes us to walk, and which consequently becomes a subject of mental contention, capable of preventing the effect of such a remedy.

There is also this inconvenience in the solitary walks of persons in feeble health, or of a melancholic temperament, that they enable such persons to deliver themselves up to those distempered ideas on which they feed; so that the result derived from it, is to return with the head and feet fatigued, and to fall into a languor worse than that from which escape was desired.

Real labour, in truth, is necessary for mankind; and the most advantageous is that which exercises equally the body and the mind. It is thus that walking may become a relaxation as salutary as agreeable, that 'the pure air, the cool shade, and the sweet perfume of flowers, pour efficaciously into the mind, with the forgetfulness of past occupations, the necessary powers to support new ones.'

RUNNING AND LEAPING

OWING to the excessive shocks which both of these exercises communicate, neither of them are very congenial to woman.

In consequence of the size of the pelvis, women are obliged to balance the centre of gravity from one side to another, in a large space, which renders these exercises very inconvenient, and which made Rousseau say, 'Women are not made for running: when they fly, it is that they may be caught. Running is not the only thing they do awkwardly; but it is the only thing they do without grace.'

Leaping might be still more dangerous than running, under many circumstances peculiar to their sex.

————————

EXERCISES OF THE FEET

BENDS IN POSITION

BENDING the hips and knees so as to turn the latter outward and rather backward, without raising the heel, and, while thus lowering the body, still keeping it perfectly erect, is an exercise which should be performed in each of the five positions. It imparts flexibility to the instep, and tends greatly to improve the balance.

In this exercise, the knees should be but slightly bent at first, and the pupil may support herself first with both hands, then alternately with each, against some fixed object, until she acquire greater power and facility. She must

PLATE XXV

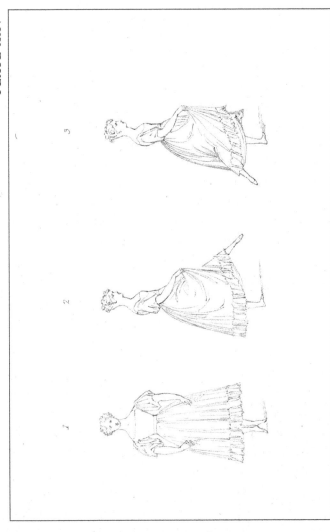

EXERCISES OF THE FEET – BENDS AND *BATTEMENTS*

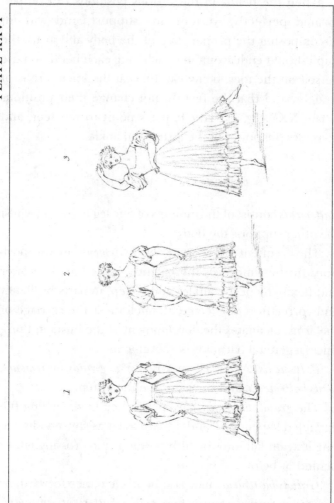

PLATE XXVI

1   2   3

EXERCISES OF THE FEET – *BATTEMENTS* AND CIRCLES

not try to raise herself by swinging the arm, which should rather be occupied in holding out the dress.

When the bends in the various positions can be performed perfectly, without any support, and without discomposing the proper state of the body and arms, the pupil should endeavour, in concluding each bend, to raise herself on the toes, being careful that the knees are kept straight, and that the feet do not change their positions (Plate XXV. *fig.* 1). This imparts point to the feet, and increases the power of the instep and ankle.

BATTEMENTS IN POSITION

Battements consist of the motions of one leg in the air, whilst the other supports the body.

The frequent practice of the *battements* in the positions further improves the balance, as well as the power and flexibility of the ankles and instep, imparts brilliancy and correctness of execution, ameliorates the carriage of the arms, facilitates the development of the bust, and produces a general harmony of movements.

Battements are of three kinds, viz. *grands battements*, *petits battements*, and *battements* on the instep.

The *grands battements* are performed by detaching the extended leg outward and upward as far as convenient, letting it again fall into the fifth position, and crossing either behind or before.

Grands battements may also be made either forward, or backward; and they are then called *battements en avant*, or *battements en arrière*.

In *battements en avant*, the right leg, with the knee

straight, is, with a jerk, raised from the fifth position into the fourth in front, as high as the left knee; keeping the toes pointed, and the foot in the same position as if on the ground (Plate XXV. *fig.* 2), and letting the leg fall back into the fifth position in front. The left leg remains steady, the knee straight, and the whole weight of the body upon it.

In *battements en arrière*, the right foot is thrown up behind in the fourth position (Plate XXV. *fig.* 3), the same circumstances being attended to as in the *battements en avant*, and great attention being paid to prevent the body inclining forward.

In performing the *battements en avant* and *en arrière*, professional dancers raise the foot much higher.

Petits battements, or *battements* on the second position, are performed in the same way, but instead of raising the leg into the air, we only detach it a little from the other leg, without letting the toe leave the ground. For this purpose, the pupil, at first supporting herself as in bending, must pass the foot into the second position (Plate XXVI. *fig.* 1), the knee being kept perfectly straight, must draw it back into the fifth position in front, pass it again into the second position, and draw it into the fifth behind, repeating this until she can perform these *battements* with correctness, ease and rapidity.

In *petits battements* on the instep, it is the hip that prepares the movements: the muscles of the hip guide the thigh in its openings, and the hip joint by its rotation directs the foot, while the knee by its flexion performs the *battements*, making the lower part of the leg cross either before or behind the other leg, which rests on the ground.

If the pupil is standing on the left foot, with the right leg

in the second position, and the right foot just touching the
ground at the toe, she must cross before the left, by bending the knee and opening again sideways; must then bend
the knee again, crossing the foot behind (Plate XXVI.
fig. 2), opening also sideways; and must so continue to do
several of these *battements*, one after the other, with increasing rapidity.

Petits battements may be first performed with one foot
entirely on the ground; but afterwards, the pupil lifts the
heel from the ground, rests entirely on the toes, and ex-
ecutes the *battements* in that position.

These *battements* have a very pretty effect, produce great
ease and suppleness in the joints just mentioned, and give
much brilliancy to the motions of the legs.

THE CIRCLES, OR *RONDS DE JAMBES*

These are performed by each foot, while the body rests
on the other, aided at first by the support of a hand. In
doing this, the body remains square to the front, and the
feet are turned well out.

In the circling limb, the knee being straight as well as
turned out, and the toe pointed downward, the circle is
begun backward or forward, passes upward as far as convenient, forward or backward as far as possible, and then
downward, so as to make a perfect circle; and this is to be
repeated several times with each limb.

To begin the circle from the outside, the pupil adopts
the same position as that in which she commences the
petits battements; and, supposing she rests on the left leg,
whilst the right, in the second position, is prepared for the

movement, she makes the latter describe a semicircle backward, which brings the legs to the first position, and she, without pausing, continues the sweep till it completes the whole circle, ending at the place whence it began.

The circle from the inside is begun in the same position; but the right leg commences the circle forward, instead of backward.

After the pupil has practised the circle on the ground, she should exercise herself in performing it in the air, holding the leg that supports the body, on the toes.

When she has acquired some facility in this, she should practise without holding, which gives uprightness and balance, essential qualities in a dancer.

Nothing more effectually ensures a good balance and supples the hip joint, than the circles.

It is equally necessary to go through the positions, bendings, *battements*, and circles, with the left foot as with the right.

PART III

COMBINATIONS OF EXERCISE

DANCING

GENERAL REMARKS

DANCING, however unscientifically it may at present be cultivated, is in reality the first of the fine arts, or that which involves the general and actual use of the muscular motions of the body, which are imitated by sculpture and painting. Scientifically practised, it is obvious that this art would not be inferior in expression to those which are merely imitative.

The dancing of the ancients was not a series of tricks with the muscles: it spoke as plainly as sculpture or painting. Hence the respect in which its professors were held, and the language of Cicero respecting Roscius.[1] Everyone is aware of the great effect which this art produced in ancient

---

1. '*Quis nostrum tam animo agresti ac duro fuit, ut Roscii morte nuper non commovetur? qui cum esset senex mortuus, tamen propter excellentum artem*

Rome, where it must have constituted a species of Acted Language. It is probable that those who practised it there were in possession of better principles than those which are now acted upon, and it is to be regretted that, at the present day, the improvement of this art is entirely left to persons unqualified for the task.

Gallini and others have so well described some of the most celebrated national dances, both ancient and modern, that I shall here follow them, with slight alteration, in a description of these.

The dances of the Greeks were figurative imitation of actions and manners. Hence Lucian requires of a dancer to be a good pantomime, and at the same time to be well acquainted with the history of the gods, or with mythology. In all the festivals of which those deities were the objects, their respective praises were sung, and those dances were executed, which represented the most striking particulars of their history; as the triumph of Bacchus, the nuptials of Vulcan, the events celebrated in the festivals of Adonis, the loves of Diana and Endymion, the flight of Daphne, the judgment of Paris, &c. The gestures, steps, movements and airs, expressed these situations.

The Cretan dance, the most ancient of all, has been described by Homer on the famous shield of Achilles.

After many other pictures, says he, Vulcan represents, with surprising variety, a figured dance, such as the ingenious Daedalus invented at Cnossus, in Crete, for the beautiful Ariadne. Young men and maidens, holding one

---

ac venustatem videbatur omnino mori non debuisse. Ergo ille corporis motu tantum amorem sibi conciliaret a nobis omnibus, &c.?'

another by the hand, dance together: the girls are habited in the richest stuffs, and wear on their heads coronets of gold: the young men appear in garments of brilliant colours. This troop[2] dance, sometimes in a round, with so much correctness and rapidity, that the motion of a wheel cannot be more equal and rapid. Now the circle of the dance breaks, and opens; then the youths, holding each other by the hand, describe in the figure an infinite number of turns and windings. This is the image of the dance which the Cretans dance at this day. The music for it is soft, and begins slow; afterwards it becomes more lively, more animated; and the young woman who leads the dance describes a number of figures and turns, of which the variety forms a very pleasing sight.

This dance of Daedalus produced, anciently, another, which was only a more complex imitation of the same subject.

In the modern Greek dance, the maidens and young men, while performing the same steps and the same figures, dance, at first, separately. After this, the two troops join, and mix so as to compose but one company of dancers. Then it is that a maiden leads the dance, taking a man by the hand; between them there is soon displayed a handkerchief or a riband, of which the couple respectively have each hold of an end. The others (and the file or row usually is not a short one) pass and repass successively under the riband. At first, they go rather slowly in a round, after which the conductress, having made a number of turnings and

2. Here the poet, from his knowledge of the dance, descriptively supplies the want of motion in the sculpture.

windings, rolls the circle round her. The art of this female dancer is to extricate herself from the maze, and to reappear on a sudden at the head of the circle, showing in her hand, with a triumphant air, her silken string, just as when she began the dance.

The meaning of the dance is obvious enough; and the description of it becomes still more interesting, when the history of its institution is known.

Theseus, returning from his expedition into Crete, after having delivered the Athenians from the heavy yoke of the tribute imposed upon them by the Cretans, himself vanquisher of the Minotaur, and possessor of Ariadne, stopped at Delos; and, after performing a solemn sacrifice to Venus, and dedicating a statue to her, which his mistress had given him, he danced with the young Athenians a dance, which in Plutarch's time was still in use among the Delians, and in which the mazy turns and windings of the labyrinth were imitated.

Callimachus, in his hymn on Delos, mentions this dance, and says that Theseus, when he instituted it, was himself the leader of it. Eustachius, on the eighteenth book of the *Iliad*, says that anciently the men and women danced separately, and that it was Theseus who first made to dance together the young men and maidens whom he had delivered from the labyrinth, in the manner that Daedalus has taught them. At Cnossus, says Pausanias, is preserved that choral dance mentioned in the *Iliad* of Homer, and which Daedalus composed for Ariadne.

At this very day, then, we see in the Greek dance, Ariadne leading her Theseus. Instead of the thread, she has a handkerchief or string in her hand, of which her partner holds the other end; and, under the string, all the rest of the dancers pass to and fro, threading it at pleasure. The tune and the dance begin at first with a slow measure; and the figure is always circular – this is the enclosure. Afterwards, the tune grows more sprightly; and the turns and windings multiplying form the maze. Ariadne, now at the head, now in the rear of the dance, turns rapidly, advances, retires, bewilders and loses herself in the midst of a numerous crowd of dancers, who follow her and describe various turns around her: Ariadne is in the midst of the maze. You would imagine her terribly perplexed how to extricate herself, when, on a sudden, you see her reappear, with her string in her hand, at the head of the dance, which she finishes in the same form as she began it. Then it is that one remembers, with pleasure, the bewildering mazes of the labyrinth, which are represented in proportion to the skill of the maiden who leads the dance, and prolongs it most with the greatest variety of turns, windings and evolutions.

Frequently, too, the young men and girls, from being intermixed, separate to form two dances, at once; that is to say, the male dancers hold up their arms under which the maidens, passing, and holding one another by the hand, dance before them; after which they return as before, and make but one row.

This is plainly the little band of Theseus, forming the like division. Here, then, is the origin of this Greek dance. Daedalus composed it at first for Ariadne, in imitation of his own famous fabric of the labyrinth. Ariadne danced it afterwards with Theseus, in memory of his happy issue out of that maze. This ancient monument has long ceased to be in existence; but the dance to which it gave rise is still preserved.

On this subject, it may be worthwhile to add, as illustrating the connexion of poetry and music with dancing, that the dance which Theseus instituted, at his return from Crete, and which he himself danced at the head of a numerous and splendid band of youth, round the altar of Apollo, was composed of three parts: the strophe, the antistrophe, and the stationary. In the strophe, the movements were from the right to the left. In the antistrophe, from the left to the right. In the stationary, they danced before the altar.

The Spartans constantly accompanied their dances with hymns and songs. Everyone knows that which they sung for the dance, called trichoria, from its being composed of three choirs, the one of children, another of young men, and the third of old. The old men opened the dance, saying, 'In time past we were valiant.' 'We are so at present,' was the response of the young. 'We shall be still more so when our time comes,' replied the chorus of the children.

Thus the art of dancing (confined at present to imitate the movements of music, which is itself often without any meaning or object of imitation) expressed, in those times, not only the actions, but the inclinations, the customs, the manners: it figured the greatest events; formed the body to strength, to agility, to dexterity, and gave graces to it: in short, it comprehended and regulated the whole art of gesture, that art nowadays so arbitrary, so uncertain, and so contracted.

The Greeks not only established academies for this exercise, but instituted games at which prizes were contended for, by excellence in the art. It was in practice among their military exercises; it took place at their entertainments, and animated their solemn festivals; even the poets recited and sang their compositions while dancing.

Plato, Aristotle, Xenophon, Plutarch, Lucian, Athenaeus, and most of the Greek authors, accordingly, treat of dancing with approbation, and even with encomia. Anacreon boasts, in his old age, that he still retains his passion for dancing. Aspasia, by her power of inspiring love, could make the sage Socrates, though advanced in years, suspend the gravity of his philosophy, to take a share in the dance. Aristides was not constrained by the presence of Plato, from dancing at an entertainment of Dionysius the Tyrant. Scipio Africanus, after the example of these great men, was not ashamed of learning and practising the dance; nor did his dignity and manliness at all suffer thereby in the opinion of the Romans. It was reckoned among the merits of Epaminondas, that he had a peculiar talent for music and dancing. But if the men valued themselves on their excelling in the art of dancing, to the women it became an indispensable accomplishment.

The cultivated dance, which is introduced in the pantomime and ballet, is a humble approach to that of the ancients, and might be rendered highly expressive.

Next to this are the modern dances to which the term National is, with some propriety, applied.

Of these, the Spanish dances, like their language, are those which, in truth of expression, approach the nearest to those of antiquity.

The fandango is the leading dance of the Spaniards, and that which stands in highest estimation. Their other dances are little more than imitations of it, and are looked upon only as second-rate.

The fandango is danced by two persons, and accompanied by castanets, instruments made of walnut-wood or of ebony. The music, in the time of $\frac{3}{8}$, is a rapid movement. The sound of the castanets, and the movements of the feet, arms and body, keep time with the greatest nicety.

In the steps of the fandango, it is the lightness, the grace, the elasticity, the balance, which are remarkable; and the more majestic movements express those feelings which mark the national character. The arms are always expanded, and their movements, in whatever direction, are always undulating.

This dance describes with vivacity the tender feeling which a beloved object inspires; and the sincerity of the avowal. The eyes, often directed towards the feet, glance over every part of the body, and testify the pleasure which symmetry of form inspires. The attitudes, the agitations of the body, the waverings, are the representatives of love, of gallantry, of impatience, of uncertainty, of vexation, of confusion, of despair, of revival, of satisfaction, and, finally, of happiness. It is by these different gradations of the passions that the nature of the Spanish dance is characterized.

The attitudes, and the graceful and voluptuous groupings of the fandango, accompanied by the cadences and thrillings of the music, have a powerful effect upon every spectator.

The lower orders in Spain accompany this dance with gross attitudes; and their extravagant movements cease only when they are completely tired out.

The bolero is a dance far more restrained, modest and dignified, than the fandango. It is executed by two persons; and is composed of five parts, namely – the *paseo* or promenade, which is a kind of introduction; the *traversias* or crossing, which alters the position of the places; the latter being done both before and after the *differencias*, a measure in which a change of steps takes place; then follow the finales; and lastly the *bien parado*, a graceful attitude, or grouping of the couple who are dancing.

The steps of the bolero are performed *terre-à-terre*: they are either sliding, beaten, or retreating, being always clearly marked.

The air of the bolero is generally in the time of $\frac{2}{4}$: there are some, however, in the time of $\frac{3}{4}$. The music is extremely varied, and full of cadences. The air or melody may be changed; but its peculiar rhythm must be preserved, together with its time and its flourishes, the latter being called also false pauses.

The original character of these dances, their pleasing and varied figure, and their expression of tender and agreeable feelings, have always obtained for them a marked preference; and, indeed, with respect to these peculiar qualities, there are few dances of other nations worthy of being compared with them. The music also that accompanies them, or, rather, that inspires them, is of a melody so sweet and original, that it finds an instantaneous welcome into the heart. The striking features of the Spanish girls, moreover, their expressive looks, their light figure, which seems formed for the dance, conspire to raise delight in the spectator. Finally, nothing can be handsomer in design, or more beautiful in its ornaments and variety of colours, than the picturesque costume of the dancers.

The Neapolitan tarantella is, of all modern dances, the liveliest and most diversified, but, like the siciliana, it possesses much similitude to the fandango. Both are, perhaps, but particularly the former, a mixture of Spanish and Italian dancing, and must have had their rise on the introduction of the Spanish style into Italy. The tarantella is gay and voluptuous, its steps, attitudes and music still exhibiting the character of those who invented it.

This dance is generally supposed to have derived its name from the tarantula, a venomous spider of Sicily. Those, it is said, who have been bitten by it cannot escape destruction, except by violent perspiration, which forces the poison out of the body through the pores of the skin; and, it is added, as exercise is the principal and surest method to effect this perspiration, music has been found to be the only incentive to the motion of the unhappy sufferers: it excites them to leap about, until extreme fatigue puts an end to their exertions; they then fall; and the perspiration thus occasioned seldom fails of effecting a cure.

The music best adapted to the performance of this kind of miracle, is excessively lively: its notes and cadences are strongly marked, and of the $\frac{6}{8}$ measure.

Love and pleasure are conspicuous throughout this dance; and each motion, each gesture, is made with the most voluptuous gracefulness. The woman tries, by her rapidity and liveliness, to excite the love of her partner, who, in his turn, endeavours to charm her with his agility, elegance, and demonstrations of tenderness. The two dancers unite, separate, return, fly into each other's arms, again bound away, and, in their different gestures, alternately exhibit love, coquetry and inconstancy. Sometimes they hold each other's hands; the man kneels down whilst the woman dances round him; again he rises; again she starts from him, and he eagerly pursues. The eye of the spectator is incessantly diverted with the variety of sentiments which they express; nor can anything be more pleasing than their picturesque groups and evolutions.

The French minuet had, probably, the same origin. The whole, however, of French dancing is too French, too vain and frivolous in its character, too offensively marked by silly affectation and ridiculous tricks, which it mistakes for expression. This is particularly remarkable in those positions called arabesques, which they Frenchify from antique basso relievos, from a few fragments of Greek painting, and from the paintings in fresco at the Vatican; and in those groups called by the same name, and formed of male and female dancers, interlaced in a thousand different manners, by means of garlands, crowns, hoops entwined with flowers, &c.

In the higher species of dancing should always be remembered the advice of Leonardo da Vinci, '*Siano l'attitudini degli uomini con le loro membra in tal modo disposte, che con quelle si dimostri l'intenzione del loro animo.*' Or, as it is more vainly and glitteringly expressed by the French poet:

> *Que la danse toujours, ou gaie ou sérieuse,*
> *Soit de nos sentiments l'image ingénieuse;*
> *Que tous ses mouvements du cœur soient les échos,*
> *Ses gestes un language, et ses pas des tableaux!*

Of the common or social dances, the most beautiful is the waltz. This dance, which came to us from Switzerland, has been modified and embellished in order to introduce into it variety.

The waltz is composed of two steps, each of three beats to a bar. Each of these two steps performs the half-turn of the waltz, which lasts during one bar. The two steps united form the whole turn, and, therefore, the whole waltz, executed in two bars. These steps differ one from the other, in such a manner, however, as to fit one into the other during their performance, so as to prevent the feet of one from touching and endangering those of the other: thus while the gentleman performs one step, the lady dances the other, so that both are executed with uninterrupted exactness.

The gentleman should support the lady by his right hand above the waist, or, if waltzing be difficult to her, he should also support her right hand by his left. The arms should be kept in a rounded position, which is the most graceful, preserving them without motion; and, in this position, one person should keep as far from the other, or make as large a circle, as the arms will permit, consistently with the rapidity of the music, so that neither may be incommoded.

The Scottish reel, which is again becoming fashionable, is a far more beautiful dance than the French quadrille.

GENERAL UTILITY OF DANCING

Dancing embraces at the same time walking, running and jumping; but it does not ordinarily enter into our systems of Gymnastics or Callisthenics, because it is taught by particular masters, and with a different intention. The ancients, however, who made all the pleasures of sense subservient to the benefit of the body, made the dance a part of their gymnastic exercises.

All active exercises are more suitable to ladies in proportion as they require less power than grace and lightness. Upon this account, the dance, beyond doubt, is, of all exercises, the most suitable to females.

This happy combination of attitudes, steps, gestures and evolutions, which is sustained by the aid of rhythm, and during which the muscles and sensibilities are employed in a manner as useful as agreeable, is indeed an unexceptionable exercise for the lower extremities; provided always that the movements are not too protracted nor performed in a style more likely to enervate than fortify the organs.

STYLE

In dancing, there may be said to be two very different styles, one that of the ballet, and another that of the ballroom. That which is beautiful in one of these, would be a defect in the other. It is the business of the professional dancer to astonish and delight; but it would be in bad taste for a lady to attempt any of those embellishments which are displayed on the stage. In society, dancing is merely an agreeable pastime; and the lady desires only to glide through the figure with ease and grace.

Private dancing requires steps *terre-à-terre*, the most simply natural postures, and a becoming grace, which add to natural charms, and heighten attractions.

Neat execution, however, ease and grace are looked for in ballroom dancing; and these must be the result of diligent practice. This practice is the more necessary, because, while it tends greatly to improvement, it serves as a valuable exercise.

OF THE FEET, &C.

In the preparation, during the performance, and at the conclusion of steps, dancers ought to stand in the fifth position, and not in the third; for the more the feet are crossed, the more brilliant is the dancing.

It is important to acquire a facility of turning the lower limbs, &c. outward.

By means of ease and power about the hip joints, the thighs will move with freedom, the knees turn outward, and all the openings of the legs be rendered easy and graceful. By practice and attention, this may be accomplished, without any painful efforts. In some steps, the hips alone are set in motion, as in *entrechats, battements tendus*, &c.

The movement of the hip is a guide to that of the knee, as it is impossible for the latter to move unless the hip acts first. The knees then should be turned outward, and rendered pliant.

It is of especial importance to acquire the power of turning the feet sufficiently outward.

It is of scarcely less importance to acquire that of bending the instep, without effort, the moment the foot quits the ground, so as to step on the toes in raising the instep. By practice, this part will habitually curve upward the moment the foot is raised from the floor, and, by a strong and rapid movement, will ensure the fall upon the toes.

Great activity about the instep renders dancing peculiarly light, brilliant and graceful.

One of the ankles must not be suffered to be habitually higher than the other: this would be a very serious defect.

Steps should be performed with minute neatness, and as closely, or in as small a compass, as possible. When rapidity is added to this, it ensures lightness and brilliance.

Each succeeding step must be well connected with the other, and all must be executed with an easy elegance.

The *moëlleux*, as the French term it, depends in a great degree on a proportionate flexion of the knees, but the instep must contribute, by its elasticity, to the elegance of the movement, and the loins must balance the frame, which the spring of the instep raises or lets down; the whole being in perfect harmony.

Defect in these qualities inevitably induces the supposition that the dancer is either unusually dull, or has never had an opportunity of obtaining proper instruction.

To attain these qualities, as well as to prevent deformity, it is necessary alternately to practise with each foot, so that both may attain an equal degree of facility and correctness.

In relation to peculiarity of form, it may be observed that, if the bust is very long, the legs may be raised a little higher than common rules prescribe; and if very short, may be kept a little lower than the usual height. By this means, the defect in the construction of the body is less apparent.

It is scarcely necessary to caution any lady against tossing the feet, lifting them high from the ground, or stamping noisily. Graceful dancing consists in gliding, not in jumping.

On the other hand, the lady must not walk languidly and carelessly, as if she had no interest in the dance. This is not only ungraceful, but has the morally bad effect of making her appear to assume the air of condescending to join in an amusement which she despises.

OF THE ARMS AND HANDS

The arms ought to be used as much as is consistent with graceful motion, in order that they may be developed equally with the lower parts of the body, and that the figure may be thus highly improved; for nothing can improve it more. As much of grace, moreover, depends on the proper position and motion of the arms, as on the execution of steps.

By professional dancers, the position, opposition and carriage of the arms, are reckoned the three most difficult things in dancing.

Great care, in the first place, must be taken not to raise the shoulders.

The arms must not be spread out too far; their general situation being a little in front of the body, in an easy semi-oval position, the bend of the elbows scarcely perceptible, and the fingers grouped and presenting a slight turn to correspond with the contour of the arms.

Ladies who are short in stature may hold the arms higher than the general rule prescribes, and those who are tall may hold them lower.

The position and carriage of the arms must be soft and easy. They must make no extravagant movement, nor must the least stiffness be allowed to creep into their motions. Care must also be taken that they are not jerked by the action of the legs, a fault sufficient to degrade a dancer, whatever perfection she may possess in other respects.

In regard to the attitude of the arms when thus free, an excellent article in the Ladies' Book, to which we are indebted for several observations, says

> Of all the movements made in dancing, the opposition or contrast of the arms with the feet is the most natural to us: to this, however, but little attention is in general paid. If any person be observed, when in the act of walking, it will be found, that when the right foot is put forward, the left arm follows, and vice versa: this is at once natural and graceful; and a similar rule should, in all cases, be followed in dancing . . . The arms should advance or recede in a natural series of oppositions to the direction of the feet in the execution of the various steps; their movements, in performing these contrasts, must not be sudden or exaggerated, but so easy as to be almost imperceptible.

This principle, though borrowed from the modern academy of painting, is altogether false.

Whenever the hands join, the arms should be kept of such moderate height as is consistent with grace.

In presenting the hand, studied attitude is productive of too much effect, and shows an inclination for display.

It is almost needless to say that, to grasp the hand of a person with whom it may be necessary to join hands, or to detain the hand when it should be relinquished, are deemed unpardonable faults.

It is almost as improper, and quite as destructive of grace, to throw one's weight upon the arms of those with whom it may be necessary to join hands.

Ladies, of course, hold their dresses with the tips of their fingers.

OF THE BUST

The shoulders must be drawn down, the chest brought forward, and the bosom slightly projected; for this confers beauty on the dancer's attitude. The waist must be held in as much as possible, the chest sustained firmly upon the loins, the upper part of the body reclined upon the hips, and the latter, as it were, expanded, in order to facilitate the motions of the legs. The whole body, however, must be well drawn up, and especially the head.

By these means, the figure at once assumes a fine form, and that firmness which is necessary to prevent its participating in the movements of the limbs.

All, however, that regards the position of the figure must be done without losing an easy and unaffected erect position.

The dancer must acquire uprightness by means of a proper balance; never letting the body depart from the perpendicular line that should fall from the pit between the collarbones through the ankles. If the dancer moves one leg forward, this pit naturally goes back out of its perpendicularity on that foot; if backward, it is thrown before; and thus it changes its place with every variation of position.

In certain attitudes, however, which dancers moment-arily throw themselves into as they spring from the ground, and also in inclined arabesques, the central line of gravity is necessarily departed from, for an instant. It must incline forward or backward, according to the position adopted.

In the performance of steps, the body must be firm and unshaken, yet perfectly pliant; its motions must be easy and always in accordance with those of the legs; and it must be characterized by a certain *abandon*, without losing the beauty of its position.

For those ladies who are round shouldered, or carry their heads too much forward, it is recommended to walk an hour, or more, every day, with a book balanced on the head, without any assistance from the hands. The lower orders of Egyptian women, we are told, are remarkable for walking majestically and gracefully, chiefly in consequence of their frequently going down to the Nile, to bring up heavy burdens of water upon their heads.

OF THE HEAD

In general, the head should be kept nearly centrally be-tween the shoulders, by the erectness of the neck. But though straight, it must never be fixed, even in the lateral direction, but must incline a little to the right or to the left, whether the eyes are cast upward, downward, or straight forward.

In general, the turn of the head will naturally be made more or less to balance the figure; so that when the great-est weight is thrown to one side, the head will generally be turned in some degree to the other; the neck inclining imperceptibly, by a continued graceful motion, in accordance with the music and the style of the dance.

Generally, the whole head should be thrown somewhat backward, though the forehead should project in a very slight degree, by correspondingly drawing the chin towards the neck.

The face must be occasionally turned to the right or left, both for convenience, and because much elegance or grace may be produced by its judicious direction, in relation to the position of the body or limbs.

The look should be neither cast down, fixed, nor wandering: it should be upon the partner, without appearing scrupulously to follow him.

The countenance should be animated and expressive of cheerfulness or gaiety, and an agreeable smile should ever play about the mouth.

OF THE WHOLE FIGURE

Rapidity, lightness, pliability, ease, harmony, elegance, are essential in a good dancer.

Rapidity is very pleasing in a dancer; lightness still more so. The former imparts brilliancy to the performance; the latter confers an aerial appearance that charms the spectator.

Pliability and a graceful *abandon* are still higher qualities in a dancer.

The keeping every part of the body, during its motions, in harmony with the rest, is a higher quality still.

The highest quality is to display all the natural elegance

that fancy can inspire in the carriage of the body, the action of the limbs, and the assumption of every attitude. No affectation must intermingle with the dance, but every attitude be natural and elegant.

Smoothness and softness in the execution of the dance, ought especially to be aimed at by ladies. They thus also show that the exercise is natural to them, and that they have overcome the greatest difficulty, namely, the concealment of art.

PECULIAR MANNER

Ladies must dance in a manner very different from gentlemen. They must delight by neat and pretty *terre-à-terre* steps, by lithsome and graceful motions, and by a modest and gentle *abandon* in all their attitudes.

The feet of women ought to be raised from the ground but very little above the method of the second position.

The manner peculiar to each individual should be in harmony with the style of her beauty.

If the features of a lady breathe gaiety and vivacity, if her shape be pretty, her dancing may be more animated, and she need not be afraid of using a style *almost* brilliant, *sissones battues, pas d'été*, &c.

If, on the contrary, a lady is of elevated stature and noble appearance, she must dance with calm elegance, or graceful dignity: slow steps and the softest movements will suit the style of her dancing. She must be careful, however, not to degenerate into stiffness, or into a contemptuous and affected negligence, like many dancers who, to give themselves an elegant and majestic air, walk or drag themselves along, and are satisfied with performing, from time to time, a few isolated steps.

Ladies who are neither very tall nor very short, and are endowed with requisite ability, may exert themselves, and may excel, in every kind of dance.

CONTINUANCE

Every lady should desist from dancing the moment she feels any difficulty of breathing; for oppression, overheating and perspiration render the most beautiful dancer an object of ridicule or of pity for the time.

It is not, however, only this momentary fatigue that should be avoided, but also lasting fatigue. When its gradual approach is felt, dancing should be left off; for it no longer affords either charm or pleasure. The steps and attitudes lose that easy elegance, that natural grace which bestow upon dancers the most enchanting appearance. The dance is nothing without grace: leave off before gracefulness leaves you.

PARTICULAR UTILITY OF DANCING

Dancing contributes greatly to improve the figure. When habitually practised, it increases the strength, the suppleness and the agility of the body. The shoulders and arms then fall farther back; the limbs become stronger and more supple; the feet turn more outward; and the walk assumes a particular character of firmness and lightness.

Dancing also renders the deportment more easy and agreeable, and the motions more free and graceful. Those, indeed, who learn to dance when very young, acquire an ease of motion that can be gained in no other way; and if a habit of moving gracefully is then acquired, it is never lost. It is owing to other causes that professional dancers are seldom remarkable for grace in any of the ordinary movements of life, and that in the performance of these they are generally constrained, formal and automatic.

As in its effect upon the muscles, dancing does not exercise any so much as those of the lower part of the trunk; they generally exhibit an evident increase at the expense of the upper part of the body and arms. This, however, is not unfavourable to female form; and the best proof of this is that this exercise produces, in men who make it their habitual practice, a great similarity in shape to women.

In professional dancers, the excess of this exercise causes the pelvis to appear large, by the prodigious development of the surrounding muscles; the neck is thin; the arms, meagre; the shoulders seem narrow, and contrast strongly with the size of the pelvis, and especially with the enormous prominence of the hips. Dancers present a formation totally different from that of smiths and porters, in whom the shoulders, chest and arms are developed at the expense of the inferior parts and lower limbs.

For these reasons, young persons, who dance a great deal, should always join with the dance some other exercise, as that of the Indian sceptres, having for its object almost exclusively the development of the shoulders and arms.

It is further observed that bad effects on the form of the foot result from overstretching its ligaments; that very few opera dancers can boast of a good instep off the stage; that when the foot is placed on the ground, the arch of the instep yields to the weight of the body, and allows the concave part of the sole to rest on the same plane with the toes; that when, therefore, these persons walk, they never rise on the toe, nor bend the foot; and that, from their habit of turning the toes very much outwards, they acquire a peculiar mode of walking.

To be useful to health, dancing must not be engaged in immediately after a meal, nor be continued whole nights, nor in places confined in proportion to the number of dancers. In these places, there is frequently a great quantity of dust, which, joined to animal exhalations, and carried with the atmospheric air into the lungs, contributes with the slightest cause, the least chill, to create irritation in the parts. These become the more serious, because young people, especially of the female sex, are very careful to conceal the commencement of these afflictions, lest they interfere with their views of pleasure.

In a physiological point of view, dancing does not differ from ordinary walking, excepting that the extensions and flexions are more quickly repeated, and that the body is every instant raised from the ground, and as if suspended in the air by the sudden straightening of the articulations. Thus, the commotions produced by this kind of exercise are stronger than those that occur in walking, and their effects on the organs contained in the trunk much more sensible. Some of the functions consequently are soon carried out of their habitual tone: the circulation becomes more rapid, the respiration more frequent, and perspiration more abundant.

Dancing is an excellent exercise for females, because it powerfully counterbalances the injurious effects of their sedentary occupations. It is particularly suited to females in whom ennui and inaction have produced habitual indisposition, to those who are of a lymphatic temperament, but more especially to young persons in whom the appearance of the phenomena peculiar to their sex and age is slow, who are subject to irregularities, and even to symptoms of chlorosis. In this case, more confidence may be put in dancing than in the list of formulas that ignorance and quackery send forth. Indeed, this exercise of the dance, to which young females resign themselves sometimes with great difficulty, forms, in addition to a tonic regimen and delicate attentions, the most suitable treatment for chlorotic affections.

There are, however, several dances that should be abandoned by very delicate women, on account of their causing too violent emotions, or an agitation which produces vertigo and nervous symptoms. Dances which require these violent shocks, and the forcible employment of the muscles, are obviously unsuitable to females, in whose movements we look for elegance instead of strength, and in whom those violent and difficult efforts, which we admire at the theatre, would create much more astonishment than delight.

Vertigo is one of the great inconveniences of the waltz; and the character of this dance, its rapid turnings, the clasping of the dancers, their exciting contact, and the too quick and too long continued succession of lively and agreeable emotions, produce sometimes, in women of a very irritable constitution, syncopes, spasms and other accidents which should induce them to renounce it.

PART IV

APPLICATION OF EXERCISES TO THE
CONDUCT OF LIFE

DEPORTMENT

A SUITABLE deportment is the proof of good education and habitual sense of order: it heightens the value of intellectual attainments, as well as constitutes a finish to beauty. As it is intimately connected with, or rather a result of, the preceding exercises, it may without impropriety be noticed here.

A dignified and graceful deportment, equally removed from frivolity and affectation, appears at first so simple, easy and natural, that it seems impertinent to lay down rules for it. The manners and style, moreover, of good society can never be acquired from books. There are, however, a few rules (subject to many exceptions and variations, without the slightest discredit either to nations or individuals) which may be termed its more material conditions. It then

PLATE XXVII

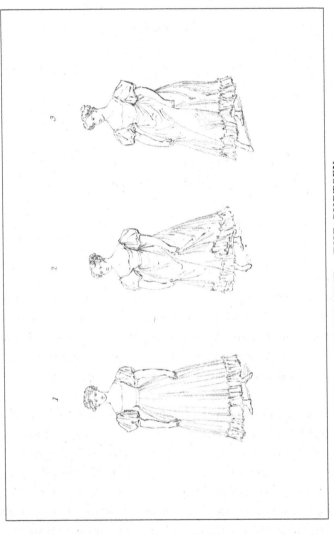

DEPORTMENT – THE CURTSEY

remains for everyone by moral disposition and by natural grace to supply the last finish.

Common sense tells us that if a friend return from a far journey, or after a long absence, we should pay the first and earliest visit; and that, in other cases, we should punctually return visits paid to us, unless we desire to avoid the society of those who have visited us.

In a visit of ceremony during winter, ladies properly quit their cloak in an antechamber, however splendid it may be. The bonnet and shawl, in a similar case, they as properly retain; and indeed, except when visiting an intimate friend, it is evident that they should not take these off, unless at the express invitation of the lady visited, or after requesting permission.

Where suitable accommodation exists, the lady visiting is duly announced; and, in any case, it is evident that to enter a room without being in some way announced, is barbarous. If there is no one to introduce the lady, she knocks gently, and waits a few seconds before opening the door, unless told to walk in. She may thus frequently avoid embarrassing situations.

There are various modes of saluting: and, in accordance with the relation of the parties, the salutation will naturally be respectful, warm, polite, affectionate, or familiar.

The curtsey,[1] to ensure ease and grace in the inevitably complex motions of the limbs, is performed as follows: When walking, the lady stops in such a manner that the weight of the body may rest upon the limb which is advanced.

---

1. A slight lowering of the person, as a mark of respect, seems natural enough, and is observed among most nations.

PLATE XXVIII

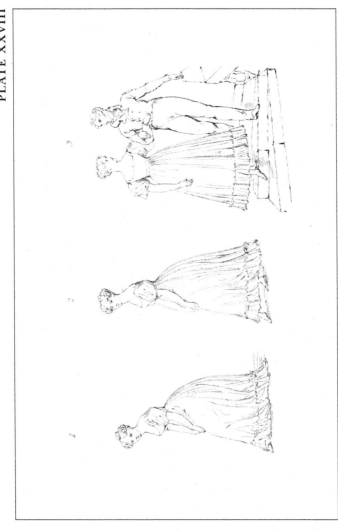

DEPORTMENT – THE CURTSEY, &C.

Then, moving the foot which is behind from the fourth hinder position, she causes it to assume successively the third and the second (Plate XXVII. *fig.* 1). Having arrived at the latter, she shifts the weight of the body upon the leg forming it, brings the other into the third position behind, and, inclining the body slightly forward, passes it immediately into the fourth behind. Preserving still the weight on the advanced leg, the knees must now bend, and the head and body further incline, and gently sink, to complete the curtsey (Plate XXVII. *fig.* 2). While rising, the weight is transferred to the foot behind (Plate XXVII. *fig.* 3), and the advanced foot is gradually brought into the fourth position. The arms should be gracefully bent, and the hands occupied in lightly holding out the dress. In walking, after the curtsey, the first step is made with the foot which happens to be forward at its completion.

A slighter form of the curtsey, more applicable to passing onward after it is made, is performed while walking, by bringing the foot of the side next to the person curtseyed to in advance at the moment of passing, throwing the weight upon it, turning the head as the person passes, bending the knees, inclining the head and body at the same time (Plate XXVIII. *fig.* 1), and then throwing, in the rise, the weight on the foot behind, and continuing the walk either by means of the foot which is advanced, or of that which is not so.

A still lighter and gayer form is to make, at the moment of passing, a slight hop on the foot furthest from the person curtseyed to, as the nearer one passes forward (Plate XXVIII. *fig.* 2), and then, keeping straight the nearer or advanced limb, which principally supports the weight, and turning the head as the person passes, to incline the body from the hips forward, and towards that person.

In entering a room where there are a number of persons, a lady, glancing round the room, naturally salutes them all at once with a more or less formal curtsey, and addresses herself especially to the lady of the house. This being done, she joins the company, and takes the first opportunity of joining also the conversation.

In the introduction of a person entering a room, the person entering is naturally first named, and next the person to whom the introduction is made, and the curtsey is reciprocal. In an accidental meeting, it is similarly the newcomer who is first named to the larger party, and then, if necessary, each of the latter in succession.

In France, where less deference is paid to rank than in England, in the case of a dinner-party, when dinner is announced, the mistress or the master of the house gets up, invites the company to follow to the dining-room, and sets them the example by passing out first. In this case, no one rises before the mistress or master of the house, and every gentleman offers his arm to a lady, to conduct her to the place where she is to sit.

A French writer accuses the English of *'the base syco-phancy of insulting age the most venerable, and genius the most admirable, by giving precedence at table to titled idiotcy,'* &c. &c. He is wrong: this was indeed once found here, as it now is in Germany; but the liberal and benevolent spirit of the age has banished such stupidities, and they are now chiefly to be seen among the cunning idiots mentioned above, or among vulgar upstarts, where their practice is the object of scarcely restrained laughter to enlightened persons.

In accepting a gentleman's arm, the lady usually passes her hand and wrist within the gentleman's forearm; but this junction of arms seems to me too complex and intimate for so short a journey, and it seems easier and more suitable for the lady to place her hand exteriorly upon the gentleman's wrist, which on his part it is certainly not less respectful properly to present. In ascending or descending stairs, she takes the side on which the steps are most regular and convenient (Plate XXVIII. *fig.* 3).

In sitting, the position of the LIMBS has considerable influence on the beauty of the figure.

The knees are generally left one by the other, scarcely separated. Though they should not be turned in, it is highly improper to turn them out in too marked a manner. It is scarcely necessary to say, that to cross them one over the other, and to embrace them with the hands joined, is deemed vulgar.

To stretch out the legs while sitting, announces conceit and pride; and to bend them up, gives a timid and frightened air.

When a lady is sitting, she generally keeps the feet but little apart, or even crossed one over the other, the right perhaps over the left, reclining on the toe and side, which certainly does not give to the foot the appearance of being less small and elegant. She in general also lowers the gown and covers the heel, so as to show little more than half the foot.

The position of the ARMS requires attention.

The general positions for the arms are about the level of the waist, never hanging down or being quite stiff, but being gently bent, the elbow a little raised, the fingers not

stretched out stiffly, but also a little bent, and partially separated, or the hands half crossed one over the other, or
placed in each other, &c. But everyone will vary all these positions from time to time, as stiffness destroys all elegance
and grace.

Several positions of the arms are vulgar: amongst others, the custom of spreading the hands separated upon the
knees; that of leaning forward and placing the arms upon
the thighs; and that of crossing them so as to place the elbows in the opposite hands. That of throwing them back
too much, and keeping them close to the side, which is
termed grasshopper-fashion, because the arms thus trussed
bear no little resemblance to the elytra of the large green
grasshopper when in a state of repose, is a mark of affectation, and is generally connected with prudery and conceit.

As to the BODY, the shoulders and chest are kept in position at the same time, but not at the expense of each other.
This is effected by straightening the back naturally, and
keeping the neck in a good position.

The movements of the body, such as quarter-turns and
half-turns, should be as natural and as easy as the involun-
tary motion of the eyelids. A lady who turns stiffly, or, as
they vulgarly say, all of a piece, is like the automaton, which
moves only by a spring.

The position of the NECK is of importance, as, from its
intermediate place, it influences both the figure and the
face. The neck inclining forward makes the back round,
makes the chin pointed, and gives the whole figure an appearance of embarrassment. Leaning backwards, it swells
in front, throws back the head in a ridiculous manner, and
fatigues the sight by its constrained attitude. Quite straight,

it wants elegance. It is, therefore, generally inclined a little
to one side, by a gentle and almost imperceptible movement, which gives it a softer character, and a more feminine
expression; but it is thus apt to acquire the character of
affectation.

Grace and ease of attitude greatly increase the beauty
of all parts of the body; whilst awkwardness and stiffness so
diminish it as to destroy its value; and affectation, preten-
sion, or negligence render it offensive.

The expression of the FACE should be under control
in all cases. Attention, astonishment, surprise, joy, and ad-
miration, carried to an excess, are as unpleasant as great
egotism, sorrow, fear, or insolence. The play of the countenance should be very marked on the stage to give force to
the dialogue, and interest to the scene represented; but this
should not be the case in society, where we should always
preserve a certain dignified respect for ourselves and for
the company.

In relation to CONVERSATION, as most people go into
society in the evening to relieve themselves from the pursuits of the morning, it is not proper to talk to anyone
upon the subject of his daily occupation. Thus we do not
talk politics with an editor, law with a barrister, or medicine
with a doctor.

It is necessary, if we go into society, to keep up a knowledge of what is going forward in the world; for, without this,
conversation is impossible.

The conversation and even the tone of the voice should
be always in accordance with the circumstances under
which the visit is paid.

In all mixed companies, it is wise to avoid remarks condemnatory of classes and professions, doctors, lawyers, or clergymen; and it is prudent to learn enough of the immediate connexions of persons present, to avoid giving pain.

Scandal was formerly the disgrace of English society: it is now felt to be base and detestable. Even satire, sneering, and mimicry are most unladylike qualifications.

Very animated conversation, a loud voice, immoderate laughter, and everything which disturbs the repose and harmony of the features, disturbs propriety and deteriorates beauty.

In relation to the management of DRESS in society, it may be observed that if the fire incommodes, a lady may, without impropriety, hold at a distance from the face a handkerchief or reticule; but it would be ridiculous to endeavour to protect clothes from the action of the fire by raising them up, doubling them back, or spreading a handkerchief over the dress.

It is also vulgar to be conspicuously careful of things which have been taken off, and impolite to manifest regret for any accident that may have befallen dress, such as spots, rents, burns. Good manners require that ladies should pay no attention to these, because that would give useless pain to others, and should hasten to turn the conversation to some other subject, thanking the mistress of the house for the anxiety she may manifest upon the subject.

Everyone has often seen stiff country ladies in full dress fold up their shawl square, put down the bonnet with care, take it up again, and replace it so as to be assured that no contact can rumple the trimming. Everyone has seen them at table spread out and then affectedly double back their gown, spread out the napkin with conspicuous care, and recommend to the servants to be careful in serving. Every-one has seen them, with troubled look, following the plate which passes over their shoulders, push back the chair when their neighbour is going to carve, and redouble their anxiety when the champagne froths up close by them.

These spectacles are by no means rare: they make us laugh, and speedily turn away the eyes, to fix them with pleasure upon those amiable ladies of perfect neatness or complete elegance who forget their dress, and exhibit an ease and bearing of the highest character. Between these two models, the choice cannot be a matter of hesitation.

The duties of a lady receiving visitors are not trifling. She is careful that all her visitors are satisfied, without, however, displaying any affectation. This task is particularly difficult when the evening is passed in dancing; for she must observe, without appearing to do so, the ladies who are not dancing, and send them partners, taking especial care that they do not observe her commission. And to fulfil properly these duties, the mistress of the house should dance but little.

If a lady is merely invited to a ball, her duties are less peremptory and less numerous, but not upon that account less indispensable. She is bound to receive, with a smiling and modest mein, all partners, whatever their age or rank. She addresses a few words with politeness to her neighbours, even though unknown to her. If they dance much, she compliments them upon their success; and if, on the contrary, they are left alone, she does not seem to perceive it, especially if she has been more fortunate: she is careful not to speak of her fatigue, or to evince an insulting compassion; and, if she can, she contributes to procure them partners,

PLATE XXIX

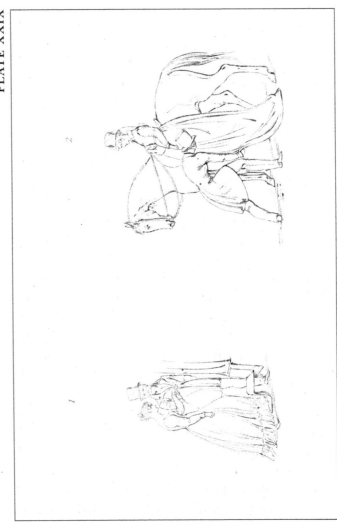

DEPORTMENT – GETTING INTO CARRIAGE, &C.

without their in any way suspecting her of the performance of such an office.

In getting into a carriage, the lady gives one hand to the gentleman assisting her, and raises her dress with the other (see Plate XXIX. *fig.* 1, in which the door and the servant who keeps it open are removed from the view).

In mounting on horseback, the lady places her right hand on the pommel of the saddle, her left foot in the right hand of the gentleman assisting her, who stoops to receive it, and her left hand on his shoulder. Then, straightening her left knee, she bears her weight on the gentleman's right hand, which he gradually raises (Plate XXIX. *fig.* 2), until she is seated on the saddle.

APPENDIX

———————

GAMES

THESE are mere trifles compared with what has already been done. It was not indeed my wish, in this work, as in the 'Manly Exercises', to teach arts of direct and practical utility in life, which are most suitable to men; but rather useful education, and more especially the preservation and improvement of beauty, and the prevention and correction of those usual tendencies to personal defect, which are inseparable from constrained or careless habits, were my objects, as here most suitable to women. Education and prevention, then, require more direct and systematic means than games. The former should, in general, be confided to teachers; the latter, with a little maternal, and, in case of actual deformity, with a little medical, guidance, may be left mainly to children themselves. It is prevention, not cure, that is the object of this work. I therefore notice but the principal of these games, and that slightly.

LE DIABLE BOITEUX

In this game, the shoulders are exercised; the rest of the arms have a stiff and awkward position; and there is little in it of an easy or graceful character.

LA GRACE

This is a new game, common in Germany, but introduced into this country from France. It derives its name from the supposed graceful attitudes which it occasions. Two sticks are held in the hands, across each other, like open scissors; and the object is to throw and catch a small hoop upon them. The game is played by two persons. When trying to catch the hoop, the sticks are held like scissors shut; and open when the hoop is thrown upward. Compared with the means already before the reader, it is as inferior as it is childish.

SKIPPING ROPE

The same remark may be made on this game, which there are several ways of practising; by simply springing and passing the rope under the feet with rapidity, once, twice, or even thrice; by crossing arms at the moment of throwing the rope; and by passing the rope under the feet of two or three, who skip at once, standing close, and laying hands on each other's shoulders.

SHUTTLECOCK AND BATTLEDORE

This game consists of striking a piece of cork covered with leather and tipped with eight or ten feathers up into the air, with a light racket covered with parchment. The object of the players is to keep the cork constantly passing and repassing in the air. It is a one-handed game, in which the right hand will always be preferred, and it is therefore peculiarly objectionable for young ladies, as ensuring that one-sidedness which is the cause of so much mischief.

BOW AND ARROW, &C.

The same strong objection may be made to this game, in which the attitude is moreover a twisted one.

———————

Bowls, nine-pins, billiards, &c. are all liable to similar objections.

———————

APPROPRIATION OF EXERCISE

EXERCISE is not equally useful in all climates.

In warm climates, heat, by calling the vital forces towards the circumference, supplies the place of exercise in many respects; and the debilitating perspirations which excite too greatly even without exercise, may render that often pernicious.

Exercise should, doubtless, be varied according to the sex of the individual.

It would, however, be a prejudicial error to suppose that females should be subjected only to passive exercise. On the contrary, the sedentary occupations of women impose upon them, more than on men, the necessity of engaging in active exercises.

Exercises should only be more moderate in woman than in man. A female, moreover, will, with advantage, use those that act upon the muscles of the chest, which her mode of life affords but few opportunities of exercising. With this view, I have already recommended, in particular, the extension motions and the Indian sceptres.

Exercise should vary according to age.

Nature announces to us, by the extreme restlessness of the infant, the pressing necessity of its organization for active exercise. In spontaneous motions, we see very young children indulge, with a kind of joy, whenever they are for an instant freed from their clothes. This is the exercise suited to their age; and it is far more salutary for them than all the motions communicated by the nurses who toss them about.

This being equally applicable to infants of both sexes, it may be added that the child should be taken out often, especially if brought up in town; but should not be kept seated on one forearm. This manner of carrying is, even in infancy, one of the causes of deviations of the vertebral column, which is still in a cartilaginous state. The mother or nurse should carry the infant on both her arms in a half reclining position, that she may give equal support to all its parts. Neither should she leave the head, which is so large in proportion to the rest of the body, to its own weight.

Above all things, it is necessary to observe that it is the movements that infants make of their own accord which are most useful to them, because the quickness of their actions should follow the vivacity of their sensations.

Medical advisers have often said that the exercise which children who cannot yet walk should be made to take, ought not to consist in being suspended by the armpits, to make them beat the ground with their feet. All the apparatus of leading-strings, by means of which nurses foolishly think to make them walk before the time appointed by nature, compresses the chest, lifts up the shoulders, frequently stops the circulation of the blood in the vessels about the armpits, and injures the respiration and circulation. The lateral deviation also of the knee-joint and ankle-joint may arise from the absurd eagerness of parents to make children walk, before their limbs are sufficiently strong to bear the disproportionate weight that the trunk presents at this age.

The exercise best suited to a child is that which it is allowed to take upon a mat or a large carpet spread upon the ground. On this species of arena, the restless creature should be allowed to throw itself about naked, and thus exercise itself in turning backwards and forwards as fancy prompts: it will thus, by successive efforts actuating generally all the muscles, soon gain the strength by which it will raise and support itself. It is similarly the liberty of running about granted to children in the country, which, in a great measure, produces that strong constitution which distinguishes them from children in towns.

In youth, active exercises are useful, in drawing into

the limbs those vivifying juices which frequently direct themselves with too much activity towards the organs of respiration and those of reproduction.

When, however, the height of a youth exceeds the usual stature, and he becomes sensibly weaker, nature evidently prescribes abstinence from violent exercise, and requires none but what may be necessary to facilitate the assimilation of the nutritive elements.

To young girls in whom an excess of liveliness and activity requires to be consumed by active and continued movements, passive exercises are not suited. It is for this age particularly that active exercises offer many advantages, and may be applied with great success. It is the period of development of all the organs, which these movements cannot but favour. It is indeed the only age at which exercise, the elements of which have been stated, is truly useful, because if deferred to a later period, they may want the activity, suppleness and skill necessary for many exercises.

In adults, exercise has the good effect of distributing, throughout the members, the vital principles, which our pernicious customs concentrate in the abdominal and cerebral organs.

In old people, exercise relieves the principal functions from the feeling of constraint which they experience, and frequently prevents those mortal strokes which at this age attack the brain.

Temperament requires to be studied in the selection of exercises.

An individual possessed of a sanguine temperament should constantly use active exercises. If sanguification or the formation of blood be very active, they may be carried so far as to produce perspiration. It is the best means of dissipating, to the advantage of the nutrition of the muscles, the excess of plethora, and superabundance of juices, which torment persons of this temperament.

Such persons ought, however, to abstain from exercises that require great efforts, on account of their predisposition to aneurysms, haemorrhages, and cerebral effusions and compressions.

Passive exercises, or those methods that gently strengthen the fibres without causing any corresponding loss, and thus induce plethora, would be unsuitable to sanguine persons disposed to haemorrhage.

Active exercises suit individuals of a lymphatic temperament, naturally dull, slow and indolent.

The ancients remarked the good effects of exercise upon girls of weak constitutions, of soft and lax texture, subject to languid maladies; and they accordingly applied exercise in the cure of many diseases that baffled the skill of the physician. The moderns have profited by their observations, and made new ones of similar tendency.

It would, however, be imprudent to subject suddenly to violent exercise young girls of feeble constitution, with soft skin, pale complexion, and light hair, which are proofs of weakness.

In persons also with soft fibres, whose narrow and feeble vessels are plunged in fat, exercise must be very moderate, in order not radically to wear out muscular forces deprived of primitive energy. If it is very violent, or is continued too long, it may then sometimes occasion adipose inflammations of the viscera.

To remedy this languishing state, their fibres should first

be braced by passive exercises frequently repeated, commencing by those which are extremely gentle. Exercise in the open air, such as carriage-riding, is particularly useful to girls of this constitution. The force and resistance of the fibres will augment in proportion as the fatty and serous plethora dissipates itself.

A nervous temperament promises superiority of the mental faculties; but it may become the source of great evils, if we do not diminish that exquisite susceptibility which sooner or later would produce them.

The general effect of exercise is to strengthen the body and counteract the early predisposition to a nervous temperament. This temperament indeed requires continual exercise. In it, there is no danger that, in strengthening the body, we may injure those faculties that seem to arise from a nervous temperament. With such constitution, no one can ever become an athlete, which, as we know, is converting mind into brute force. Nervous girls, then, should be strengthened; it will prevent them becoming invalids; it is certain they will remain clever.

A physician accordingly observes that, in strengthening the animal economy by exercise, we get rid of the nervous irritability, the sickly sensibility, which is the offspring of luxury, and parent of vapours, hysterics and hypochondria, as well as of the fatal practices which attack the sources of life, and which commence at the age of puberty and often sooner. By strengthening the muscles, exercise moderates this vicious sensibility. Exercise produces lassitude, and lassitude sleep; and when a person sleeps soundly, she will not be awakened by the fancies of a disordered imagination.

Passive, mixed, and moderately active exercises suit a

bilious temperament, characterized by dryness and extreme rigidity of fibre. The individual should use moderate and sustained exercise, fit rather to regulate than accelerate the march of functions already too rapid.

Particular dispositions also require particular exercises. One cannot endure the motion of the most easy carriage; another suffers from that of a boat; a third finds it impossible to ride on horseback, &c. It is sometimes desirable to combat these dislikes, but we must not obstinately endeavour to surmount them, when they appear determined: it is better, in such a case, to discontinue the exercise disliked: and frequently another, even more active, will not produce the same inconvenience.

The habits previously contracted should not be overlooked in advising as to exercise. A young girl whose condition is sedentary, should not be subjected to such exercise as a young man who is generally actively employed. The best application of gymnastics, is that which conducts the pupil gradually from the most gentle exercise to the most active.

Without speaking of acute maladies, in which muscular action is always hurtful, there are different states of the body in which the utility of exercise is very doubtful: there are even some in which, by the nature of its direct effects, it can do only ill. Such is the case with young girls who may be affected with predisposition to apoplexy, asthmatical diseases, &c.

It is evident that in general passive exercises only should be had recourse to in case of sickness and indispositions, because spontaneous movement might then be more or less injurious.

Exercise, however, if properly directed, is extremely beneficial in convalescence. The recovering patient who cannot yet walk across her chamber, should be carried or wheeled in an easy chair, until she can support the motion of a carriage.

Many chronic afflictions are favourably influenced by exercise; but of course it must be taken under the precautions we have mentioned for convalescents. In these cases and others analogous, where passive exercises are useful, it rarely happens that the use of active exercises is successful.

The same does not hold in scrofulous cases, where debility, paleness, and want of elasticity indicate the necessity of motions as active as the strength will admit. It is probable that these diseases, so common in infancy and youth, will be very rare in children who are regularly trained to exercise.

It is at the age of puberty, especially, that exercise has an influence remarkably favourable over the diseases to which young girls are subject.

Where girls have been, from their infancy, habituated to suitable exercises, the phenomena peculiar to them make their appearance much later than when they have been brought up in idleness and luxury, and consequently at a period when the constitution has more power to resist the accidents that then occur.

It is strikingly the reverse, where girls have lived in the midst of pleasures, where night is turned into day, and spent many of these nights in dances, where the salutary effect of motion is counteracted by the unhealthy effect of large numbers in a circumscribed space, where there is scarcely room to breathe a heated and corrupted air. Exercise like this, far from strengthening the body, produces only a momentary excitement, which increases vicious sensibility, and lays the foundations of a diseased maturity. In some cases, where the languid and inert state of the organs requires rousing, exercise, by exciting the action of the principal organ, brings on the desired event, and facilitates its periodical return, and thus brings back, with more certainty than any medicinal means, health, strength and beauty.

GUIDANCE OF EXERCISES

In regard to the time for exercise in the open air, the morning is usually directed to be chosen in summer, and the middle of the day in winter.

This rule is not necessary as to exercise taken under cover; but violent exercise should never be suffered in summer, at that part of the day when the heat is most powerful.

The state of the body is a circumstance not to be neglected.

Active exercises should not be indulged in, except when digestion has been finished, because the animal organization does not properly perform several actions at the same time.

Very moderate exercises, such as walking or carriage-riding, may be indulged immediately after a meal. Still it is not proper for persons who are in a state of perfect health, and in the constant habit of using bodily exercise, to practise these exercises, however moderate, in the idea of aiding in the accomplishment of any kind of function of life.

Passive exercise is generally most favourable to digestion.

Meals, on the other hand, should never be taken immediately after violent exercise. The stimulus produced by them in the economy, deranges the order of the vital movements, and for a time deprives the stomach of the strength requisite for its function.

In a perspiration, it is not possible, without some danger, to return to passive exercise, during which there is inactivity. Similar precautions are still more necessary at certain periods.

It is also advisable not to commence these exercises without satisfying any demands of nature that might become troublesome or dangerous.

The clothes should be made of strong materials, not so expensive as to make it of consequence if they should be spoilt in the exercise. They should not be so tight as to constrain the motions, nor so large as to embarrass by their looseness. They should contain nothing capable of hurting. The shoes should be large. No band should confine the body or limbs: the shoulder-straps of stays should be loosened, and it is better to wear neither sash, nor garters. Everything that may prevent freedom of action should be rejected.

The choice of a place for exercise, is by no means a matter of indifference. Other things being equal, the body will receive more salutary influences from exercise taken in the open air, in the middle of a field, in a pleasant, agreeable country. Independently of its effects upon the mind, the breathing of a more pure and animating air and the exciting action of the light, produce an effect which would be in vain expected in a confined place, and especially in a room or courtyard.

There are, however, cases in which exposure to the open air might produce some inconvenience, and in which it is desirable to choose such exercise as can be taken in a close place.

Accordingly, a place for exercise cannot offer all the advantages to be expected from it, except it be sufficiently spacious not only to permit a variety of games, but to allow the means, according to circumstances and necessity, of exercising either in the open air, or in an enclosed space, and in all kinds of situations.

It is of the very highest importance to bear in mind that ACTIVE EXERCISES SHOULD BE SO DIRECTED AS TO KEEP UP THE REGULAR ACTION OF ALL THE MUSCULAR PARTS AND TO EXCITE THE ACTION OF THOSE WHICH ARE LESS DEVELOPED. *It is the attention bestowed on this precept which is the means of preventing those deviations of the vertebral column, that may be observed amongst the majority of young girls.*

Active exercises should be proceeded with gradually; those that require the employment of great strength should not be commenced till custom has rendered easy those that require less.

Active exercises should be proportioned to what can be spared by the other organs in favour of muscular action; for violent and continued movements would soon produce disorder. Under the influence of such exercise, the palpitations of the heart are immoderate, the breathing becomes difficult, the heat excessive, the perspiration streams over an inflamed skin, digestion is deranged, the body loses what it does not regain, langour and debility are felt, and falling away takes place without the texture of the organs becoming stronger.

No general rule can be laid down for the duration of exercise. What might be easy for some would fatigue others. We must therefore consult the age, strength, temperament and habits, so as not to require violent and long-continued efforts from one incapable of supporting them.

The best rule is to stop before we feel fatigued, otherwise we risk the chance of weakening, instead of strengthening. Motions sufficiently violent to produce a painful state of fatigue, cannot be continued without efforts which must be continually increased, and will speedily produce a violent excitement and disorder of the functions.

Exercise, to be useful and salutary, should be frequent rather than violent.

It is not necessary that exercise should be the object of a scrupulous calculation. It is better to consult present taste or feeling than chimerical ideas of order and regularity. A life too measured out, by subjecting her who assumes it to the influence of habit, exposes her more to the attacks of disease. Change is even necessary to prepare us for violent shocks.

When the exhaling vessels of the skin act powerfully in consequence of violent exercise, and perspiration bedews every part of the body, it must not be suddenly stopped: the animal economy requires this, in order to get rid of too great heat; and if it were suddenly suspended, the feverish action occasioned by exercise, finding no longer means of a salutary crisis, through cutaneous exhalation, might injuriously influence the viscera, and produce there that fluxion which was going off by the pores of the skin. In this case, those organs, which, in consequence of any predisposing cause, were most disposed to irritation, would be the first affected.

To obviate this inconvenience, and give time for the fluxion we are speaking of to diminish, and cease only when the object of nature is attained, it is prudent to resume clothes, if they have been diminished during the exercise, or if not, and they are impregnated with moisture, to change them for others.

Everyone knows that, in this state, no part of the body should be exposed uncovered to cold, and especially to a draught: drinking a quantity of cold water, or placing the hands or feet in cold water when the heat is abating, is still more carefully to be avoided. These precautions, which seem most necessary in winter and cold weather, must not be neglected in summer, when heat and perspiration are more easily excited.

In no case, after violent exercise, should the exerciser remain in a state of total inaction. After violent exercise, the pupil should indulge in a more gentle sort, so as gradually to allay the excitement raised. If she prefers resting inactive, she should return to some warm place to dry herself, rub the skin gently, and assume a change of linen.

FINIS

MEDICAL TESTIMONIALS

***

LETTER FROM DR BIRKBECK TO THE AUTHOR

38, Finsbury Square; 11 Dec. 1835

MY DEAR SIR,

To promote and to regulate the exercise of young ladies, are objects not less important than difficult; and I am delighted to see an attempt made by the author of 'Manly Exercises', for their accomplishment.

With your general views regarding female development, which are clear and well expressed, I thoroughly agree: and I am not less gratified by what you have stated respecting the necessity of early freedom from all restraint of a personal kind, of equality of action and position, and of constant, appropriate, well regulated exercise, to the production alike of grace, of health, and of vigour. You have contributed materially, I am persuaded, to prevent the occurrence of unequal enlargement of muscular parts, the first and slightest species of deformity; and the still more serious deviations from the correct form of the body, which occur when that curious and beautiful mechanical fabric the spine, becomes deranged. The means which you have proposed for the correction of such casualties when they do occur, are excellent; and will, I trust, quickly supersede the use of all those inconsistent and unscientific expedients, which under the pretext of producing support and extension, augment the essential cause of deformity, by crippling the natural actions, overloading the weakened frame, and exerting much unequal and painful pressure.

The modes of action which, in your work, you have proposed as exercises for ladies, are good; and some of them are interesting and amusing. It has occurred to me often to observe, that for the recommendation of suitable and sufficient exercise, it was not enough powerfully to display its ultimate importance to the well-being of the individual; it was necessary to secure its adoption, to render it attractive likewise. Hence, the advantage of dancing; and hence the advantage of the Indian Exercise, which by its elegance, variety, and moderation, will, I doubt not, when your work has been extensively circulated, become a general favorite. Indeed, I am not acquainted with any modifications of action, which in conferring grace, facility, and power, can be compared with the Indian Exercise.

That in this new endeavour to improve the physical condition of our species – and in this instance, unquestionably the most interesting portion – I hope you may be eminently successful, after what I have written upon the subject, cannot be doubted: and I remain ever, my dear Sir,

Very sincerely and faithfully yours,

GEORGE BIRKBECK

To Donald Walker, Esq.

LETTER FROM DR COPLAND TO THE AUTHOR

Bulstrode Street; 10 Dec. 1835

DEAR SIR,

I have been very much pleased by the perusal of your book on the *Exercises for Ladies*, &c.

I agree with you in the opinion, that the universal and perpetually operating cause of deformity in young ladies is the '*one-sidedness*' with which nearly every action in common life is performed. Of the safety and efficacy of the exercises you recommend I have no doubt. The Indian sceptre exercise is the most efficient and most graceful of any hitherto devised.

Upon the whole, I esteem the exercises described to be the best calculated, of any means that have come to my knowledge, to prevent deformity, to remedy it in most cases, and to promote a healthy physical development.

I am, dear Sir, yours truly,

JAMES COPLAND, M.D. F.R.S. &C.

To Donald Walker, Esq.

AUTHOR'S NOTE

_____

INNUMERABLE parents have watched with anxiety the ostensible operation of the causes producing deformity in their daughters. Few have imagined that these causes are almost as palpable as their effects, that they are their peculiar modes of performing nearly every act of their lives!

But this is less surprising than that medical writers, so far as I am acquainted with them, should, with regard, for instance, to the most universal of these deformities – lateral curvature of the spinal column – have generally failed to give simple and lucid views, in due succession, of the structure and functions of the parts chiefly affected, of the causes acting upon them, of the uniformity with which these exert one lateral action, of the one-sidedness which characterizes all of them, and of the clear indication of the means of prevention, namely, a little othersidedness, which this knowledge of the cause presents.

Under such circumstances, it is not wonderful that the teachers of exercises, who are generally destitute of physiological knowledge, should have hitherto proposed inadequate and ridiculous means – exercises which, in almost every instance, have been either uselessly severe, or unmeaning and frivolous.

The materials, however, on this important subject have been almost as ample as could be desired. Nothing has been wanted, but a very little analytical enquiry, and an orderly disposition of well-known facts.

I pretend, accordingly, to have done no more as to existing materials than to select from others the most striking of these facts, not disguising my obligations even by verbal changes, but once for all acknowledging them, as I now do, and to have put these facts in a somewhat clearer point of view, to have, in fact, employed upon them the little analysis and generalization they seemed to require, to have more clearly established the truth that this one-sidedness is the general cause of deformity, and that its prevention requires an equal and similar use of the other side.

Beside this, however, I have endeavoured to contribute my full share of new materials I believe to have the claim of perfect novelty.

D. W.

1 November, 1835

N.B. I beg to refer to Mr Goadby, of No. 97, B. in the Quadrant, Regent Street, as being, of all these exercises, by far the best teacher with whom I am acquainted.

Of the same gentleman, or of the Publisher, Mr Hurst, 65, St Paul's Church Yard, may be had the Indian sceptres, or whatever else may be required in these exercises. Ladies, however, who from any cause find it difficult to procure sceptres, may have made, by any carpenter, two pieces of plain and smooth wood, about two feet long (including the narrower portion for a handle, to terminate in a knob) and loaded with lead at their lower and larger extremity, so as to furnish any convenient weight, as two, three, or four pounds.